Toxic Trauma

David J. Baker

Toxic Trauma

A Basic Clinical Guide

Second Edition

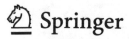

David J. Baker
SAMU de Paris
Hôpital Necker—Enfants Malades
Paris
France

ISBN 978-3-319-82216-7   ISBN 978-3-319-40916-0   (eBook)
DOI 10.1007/978-3-319-40916-0

This Springer imprint is published by Springer Nature
The registered company is Springer International Publishing AG
The registered company address is: Gewerbestrasse 11, 6330 Cham, Switzerland

This book is dedicated to all those who have suffered toxic trauma and to those who have cared for them, in war and in peace.

Foreword

One of the most testing problems an emergency physician or clinical toxicologist can face is posed by a seriously ill or unconscious patient who appears to have been exposed to some toxic substance and whose clinical condition is rapidly worsening. Whether the identity of the substance is known from the clinical history or circumstances of exposure, or is unknown, it is likely that immediate treatment to support vital physiological functions will be needed. Contrary to popular opinion, specific antidotes are few in number and, in any case, cannot be given until the identity of the toxic substance, or substances, has been discovered. This may take some time, and time is a luxury seldom enjoyed by the emergency physician. As soon as one steps outside the range of drugs and chemicals too often chosen by those with suicidal intent, the range of toxic substances to which the patient may have been exposed becomes vast and includes materials of animal, plant and bacterial origin in addition to the innumerable toxic chemicals produced by man. A special case of the latter is provided by radioactive materials. In addition, though of less immediate importance to the physician, exposure may have been accidental or may reflect not suicidal but homicidal intent. One example of homicidal intent is provided by a terrorist attack involving the release of toxic chemicals and exposure of the civilian population. The 1995 attack on the users of the Tokyo subway and the attack on civilians in Damascus in 2013 provide examples of such activity. Such incidents pose a further burden on the emergency physician: not one but many patients who may be critically ill as a result of exposure to an unknown chemical or chemicals may have to be dealt with simultaneously. That anybody should be deliberately exposed to toxic chemicals is appalling; that physicians should be ill-prepared to deal with the clinical consequences of such attacks would be irresponsible folly.

Dr. Baker has addressed these problems in this new edition of Toxic Trauma. He has developed and refined the concepts of supportive and specific therapy by defining a series of toxidromes (clinical syndromes associated with exposure to toxic substances) that characterise the effects of a number of groups of toxic materials. These toxidromes are, in my view very sensibly, defined in terms of the pathophysiological effects of groups of chemicals: understanding the pathophysiology leads to rational therapy. He has gone beyond mere definition: he has produced clear and concise advice on clinical measures needed to deal with the effects of such groups of toxic materials. His thinking is based on his wide experience of clinical toxicology and on his special expertise in the field of the toxicology of chemical warfare agents. It is in the latter field that the problems of dealing with chemical casualties are met at their most acute, and lessons learnt in this field can hardly fail to be of importance when civilian casualties of terrorist attacks have to be treated, indeed they should be remembered when any patients exposed to toxic chemicals are treated.

Prof. R.L. Maynard, CBE FRCP
Honorary Professor of Environmental Medicine
University of Birmingham, UK

Preface to the Second Edition

The object of the first edition of this book was to provide practical guidance to emergency medical responders faced with the problem of managing casualties from chemical agents, either accidental or as an act of warfare or terrorism. This was placed within the framework of the concept of toxic trauma, which considers that injury to the body as a result of toxic exposure should be regarded as part of the whole spectrum of trauma, which includes both the blunt and penetrating forms of physical trauma.

This approach appears to have been well received by readers of the first edition, judging from reviews and personal feedback to the author. This new edition of *Toxic Trauma* follows essentially the same structure as the first, but a number of sections have been expanded and there is a new chapter, which considers the place of chemical agents as part of the chemical, biological, radiological and nuclear (CBRN) classification of hazards which are often termed 'weapons of mass destruction'. The CBRN grouping, the types of trauma caused and the necessary responses are often poorly understood by medical, paramedical and nursing personnel who are only infrequently required to deal with casualties from each of the CBRN hazards. In reality, CBRN agents, while having some common characteristics, cause trauma in very different ways which require an adapted medical response. Radiation injury and radioactivity, in particular, are not always well understood by emergency medical responders, and the new final chapter attempts to provide a simple introduction to fill this gap.

Since the appearance of the first edition, toxic trauma from deliberate exposure to chemical warfare agents has continued in the Syrian Civil War, causing many thousands of casualties. The fear of further use of chemical weapons by terrorist organisations continues, and thus readiness to deal with chemical casualties in the urban civil setting remains more important than ever. In industrial and domestic settings, the accidental release of toxic chemicals continues and no hospital department can afford not to prepare for such incidents, both in daily practice and as part of disaster-response planning. The hazards of toxic trauma remain therefore as real as ever, and I hope that the new edition of this book will help to inform and to prepare responses accordingly.

I would like to acknowledge colleagues who reviewed the first edition and provided many helpful comments, notably Dr. Samuel Delerme, Dr. Michael Nurok and Prof. Robert Maynard, who has kindly provided a foreword to the present edition. I would also like to thank the editorial team at Springer Verlag for all their help and support. Finally, I would like to thank my wife and colleague Dr. Marian Barry for her invaluable help with reading and correcting the proofs.

I hope that the new edition of *Toxic Trauma* will prove to be essentially practical and readable by the non-specialists for whom it is written and will encourage more interest in what has in the past been a rather remote area of practice for many.

Paris, France   David J. Baker

Preface to the First Edition

The past 30 years have seen the development of a rational and comprehensive approach to the management of physical trauma in response to a steady world-wide increase in the numbers of those injured in both peace and war. In civil emergency medicine, there has been increasing experience of the management of physical trauma from road traffic accidents, natural disasters such as earthquakes together with gunshot wounds and blast injury from terrorist improvised explosive devices, while continuing wars around the world have meant that a new generation of military medical personnel has had extensive experience of modern trauma management.

Systematic training courses such as the US College of Surgeons Advanced Trauma Life Support (ATLS™) and other national programmes have been developed and are widely taught around the world. Trauma management has become a standard part of the training of surgeons, emergency medical physicians, anaesthetists and other medical and paramedical specialities, and an early systematic approach has had considerable impact on the clinical outcome.

In contrast, the management of casualties following exposure to toxic chemicals has not received quite the same attention, although evidence shows that both military and civil pre-hospital and hospital medical personnel are increasingly likely to be required to treat such cases. In the civil setting, the risks are increasing, as is public awareness and fear of chemical exposure. Nearly a century after the first large-scale use of chemicals in warfare, the threat of chemical exposure still remains and has now been extended to deliberate release on civil populations by terrorists. In addition, accidental releases of toxic industrial chemicals have produced catastrophic consequences, particularly in developing countries where medical care may be limited.

The management of exposure to toxic chemicals goes beyond the relatively familiar emergency room situation of accidental or deliberate ingestion of poisons and requires a medical approach that ensures both a rapid and effective response for the patient and also protection of the responders against the secondary effects of the causative toxic agent to ensure they do not become casualties themselves. Accidental release of hazardous toxic materials (HAZMAT) is managed according to international guidelines and, following the precedent set by physical trauma specialist, training courses such as the Advanced Hazmat Life Support Course (AHLS™) have been developed. However, participation in these and experience of the management of casualties of toxic releases are not as widespread as for physical trauma.

Individual poisoning is most familiar by ingestion but exposure to toxic chemicals, with entry to the body through other routes such as respiratory system and the skin, can potentially affect all the systems of the body. In addition, there are a number of identified pathways of pathophysiological damage that are convergent with those of conventional physical trauma. Respiratory and cardiac arrest together with organ failure may be a terminal event following both physical trauma and exposure to toxic chemicals, and in severe cases intensive care is required in both situations.

From the overall standpoint of injury management, the systematic medical management of exposure to toxic substances may be viewed as part of a spectrum of the various forms of physical trauma and which may be termed 'toxic trauma'. The management of toxic trauma goes beyond the conventional clinical toxico-logical management of ingested poisoning and links together other specialities who are individually concerned with the management of toxic effects on specific body systems, notably neurological, respiratory, cardiac, opthalmological and dermal. In addition, the concept of toxic trauma, rather than poisoning *per se*, serves to underline the potential danger to medical responders from the same toxic substance that has caused the primary injuries which is not often a problem in the emergency room following poisoning by ingestion or envenomation.

There is a widely held view among the general public that injuries from the mass release of chemical agents, which are often regarded as being 'weapons of mass destruction', cannot be treated and will be inevitably fatal. This has given rise to a fear of chemical exposure which is out of proportion to the potential injury. A positive approach by medical professionals and the integration of the manage-ment of toxic trauma into other trauma management will do much to restore public confidence and order in the event of a terrorist attack or other toxic release with the realisation that while chemical agents may cause mass injuries, these can be pre-vented or treated with a prepared and coordinated medical response.

The object of this book was to provide a basic understanding and practical guidance to emergency personnel and others faced with the possibly unfamiliar situation of having to manage individual or mass chemical casualties as part of their work in a civilian ambulance service or hospital. The text will consider the nature of the hazards faced and the practical management of persons exposed to chemicals and to toxins (which although of biological origin behave as chemicals in terms of their effects and transmission).

The individual chapters will consider the development and classification of chemical toxic agents, how exposure can occur and how medical personnel should be involved in its management. Subsequent sections consider the nature of toxic trauma and the pathophysiology processes involved, together with a systematic approach to early and continuing management. In addition, examples of incidents are presented. The aim of this guide is to help emergency medical and paramedical personnel become familiar not only with the management of the victims but also how to operate safely within potentially contaminated areas to prevent them also becoming secondary casualties from a chemical release.

World wide, there is a continuing risk of exposure to chemical agents from both accidental industrial discharges and deliberate release of chemical warfare agents and toxins as part of chemical warfare or terrorist activity. In the military and terrorist contexts, chemical agents are grouped together with biological, radiological (radioisotopes) and nuclear weapons (CBRN) in terms of management. In practice, however, the management of chemical exposure is very different from the management of infection with biological agents and exposure to radiation. Thus, the management of biological, radiological and nuclear explosive exposure will not be considered in this text. These can cause physical trauma and systemic effects, but the management of infection and radiation injury is the subject of many specialised texts. There are also many detailed clinical toxicological texts available concerning the management of individual poisoning which this book will not attempt to duplicate.

The literature about exposure to toxic chemicals in peace and war is vast and usually too detailed for the reading time available to busy emergency medical responders. Equally, there are a number of short guides to the management of hazardous materials releases which do not explain the pathophysiology and most importantly the details of life support measures and specific therapy from the standpoint of a trained physician. To attempt to bridge this gap, each of the following chapters provides a synopsis of the current thinking, concerning the nature and management of toxic trauma based upon detailed published information in specialised texts and the author's personal experience over a number of years in the field. A selection of suggestions for further reading is provided for each section which will provide further detailed information for those requiring it. Specific referencing of the text has been avoided for simplicity of reading. However, the suggestions for further reading have been selected because the texts contain lists of essential references from a wide range of medical and scientific fields that have provided the basis of our knowledge about the effects of chemical exposure.

In particular, I have drawn upon the detailed and authoritative volume on chemical warfare agents which a is part of the continuing series of publications that forms the monumental US Army Textbook of Military Medicine. This and other more specialised texts will perhaps be beyond the reading time available to non-specialists, and I hope that my distillation of information will be accurate and appropriate.

The object of this book was to provide a concise clinical guide to the nature and management of toxic trauma which can be used to aid preparation and responses to releases of chemical agents. Hopefully, it will help to promote confidence and a positive approach to chemical casualty management among those who find themselves in what may be an unfamiliar situation with possibly little or no advance warning and will promote an integration of toxic trauma into a comprehensive approach to the overall management of trauma.

David J. Baker

Contents

About the Author

David J. Baker studied medicine at St. Bartholomew's Hospital, London and served for 20 years as a medical officer in the Royal Navy, specialising in anaesthesia and neurotoxicology. Later he worked as a consultant in anaesthesia for the Paris emergency medical service (SAMU) at the Necker University Hospital and advised on the management of mass toxic incidents. From 2004, he also worked as a consultant medical toxicologist for the Centre for Radiation, Chemical and Environmental Hazards of the United Kingdom Health Protection Agency. Since 2005, he has worked as a visiting professor at Harvard Medical School and as a visiting senior lecturer in medical toxicology at King's College, London. Currently he is working on the management of pulmonary injury following toxic agent inhalation and on the provision of early ventilatory support following toxic respiratory failure. He has lectured in over 40 countries around the world and is the author of numerous journal articles, monographs and textbook chapters. He has been a Board Member of the World Association for Disaster and Emergency Medicine and has consulted for the World Health Organisation and the International Committee of the Red Cross.

Chapter 1
Introduction

Abstract Trauma may be defined as the effects of external harmful forces that disrupt both the structure and function of the body and is familiar in its various forms such as penetrating, blunt, crush and thermal trauma. The actions of toxic chemicals on the body can be integrated into the various forms of physical trauma as what might be termed 'toxic trauma'. Toxic trauma can be defined broadly as the disruption of somatic systems and their function by exposure to a toxic chemical. Toxic chemical agents injure through a variety of routes of entry into the body and by affecting several somatic systems. An understanding of the pathophysiogical processes involved is essential to management as is a systematic approach to clinical management that has been the keystone of modern physical trauma management. This chapter considers an integrated approach to trauma and its clinical advantages for management and improved outcome.

1.1 Trauma: A Worldwide Epidemic

Human life is constantly threatened by injury from a number of external physical hazards. The management of injury, once seen widely only in battle, has now become a major part of the work of emergency physicians worldwide. Trauma is a growing problem around the world which places a heavy burden on health systems. It is familiar in many forms in both war and peace, and the first stages in its systematic management date from the Napoleonic Wars. In civil life, trauma has been steadily increasing from the increase in road traffic accidents, natural disasters and the increasing use of improvised explosive devices by terrorists. However, the growth of physical trauma has been accompanied by a parallel increase in the number of persons exposed to toxic chemicals. Casualties from such exposures are less familiar to emergency medical teams than those from physical trauma.

Around the world, in civil as well as in military settings, emergency care has to be given to individual or mass casualties who present at a hospital after a life-threatening event. Usually, this care is required for victims of physical trauma, but there is also an increasing possibility of having to deal with casualties from a

© Springer International Publishing Switzerland 2016
D.J. Baker, *Toxic Trauma*, DOI 10.1007/978-3-319-40916-0_1

toxic release, which can have grave consequences both for the patient and for the responding medical services. In some cases, chemical releases may be accompanied by explosion or fire-producing casualties who are affected by both physical and toxic injuries. There is therefore a need to approach the management of trauma from both its physical and toxic causes.

1.2   Physical Trauma

Physical trauma may be defined as the effects of external harmful forces that disrupt both the structure and the function of the body. Such trauma has been a familiar feature of life since prehistoric times up to the present day, in both war and peace. Overall, its incidence is increasing and it places a great strain upon health systems worldwide (Box 1.1). Penetrating wounds, earlier from spears and swords and later from guns, are familiar to most people around the world, whether through direct experience or from television pictures. This is one form of physical trauma. Equally familiar are the effects of crushing trauma from earthquakes and the collapse of buildings. Explosions cause blast and blunt physical trauma, which is also familiar from road traffic incidents, falls or violent assaults. In addition to blunt and pene-trating trauma, thermal trauma from burns or extreme cold places a continuing burden on health systems around the world.

Box 1.1 The Scale of Physical Trauma Worldwide
Injuries resulting from traffic collisions, drowning, poisoning, falls or burns and violence—from assault, self-inflicted violence or acts of war—kill more than 5 million people worldwide annually and cause harm to millions more. They account for 9 % of global mortality and are a threat to health in every country of the world. For every death, it is estimated that there are dozens of hospitalizations, hundreds of emergency department visits and thousands of doctors' appointments. A large proportion of people surviving their injuries incur temporary or permanent disabilities.

Source World Health Organization, 2013 http://.who.int/topics/injuries/en. Accessed 21/07/13

In all its forms, physical trauma has immediately recognisable consequences on both body form and function, which start a short period after the harmful action. Injury of this type is defined as having a short latency although many harmful consequences may occur later following the initial injury. These may arise directly from the injury or as a result of severe haemorrhage and shock which can cause non-reversible damage to body systems. Examples of easily recognisable short-latency physical trauma are fractured bones with deformity, haemorrhage and head injury, which causes loss of consciousness. In some cases such as explosive injury, there may be major injuries such as traumatic amputation. As a result of media coverage, the effects of trauma, previously seen only by those who had lived near or through the violent episode, for example, in warfare, are now familiar to many millions of people around the world on a daily basis.

1.3   Responses to Physical Trauma

Trauma places a heavy burden on health systems around the world, particularly in countries which have the least developed resources. Although doctors and surgeons have been treating physical trauma in war and in peace for thousands of years, it is only over the past few decades that planned responses to trauma, such as the US Advanced Trauma Life Support (ATLS™; Box 1.2) programme and its modification for use in the military sphere, have been developed, which adopt a systematic approach to the initial and continuing management. Such systems have produced a more rational approach to the early problems of physical trauma, and this has made a great difference to survival rates.

> **Box 1.2 Advanced Trauma Life Support**
> A new approach to the provision of care for individuals suffering from major life threatening injury started in 1978, the year of the first ATLS™ course. In January 1980, the American College of Surgeons (ACS) introduced the ATLS™ course in the USA and abroad. Canada joined the ATLS™ programme the following year. In 1986, several countries in Latin America joined the ACS Committee on Trauma and introduced the ATLS™ programme in their region. Now, ATLS™ is available in nearly 60 countries.
>
> Since the ACS Committee on Trauma has taught the ATLS™ course to more than 1 million doctors in more than 50 countries, other countries have developed their own approaches to teaching the management of physical trauma with the production of a global systematic approach to the problem.
>
> *Source* http://www.facs.org/trauma/atls/history.atm/

1.3.1   The Historical Timeline of Systematic Trauma Management

Dominique Jean Larrey, Napoleon's surgeon-in-chief and Baron Pierre-François Percy (Box 1.3) were the first surgeons to understand the need for a rapid response to trauma and for prioritising treatment. It became clear during the nineteenth and twentieth centuries that mortality from physical trauma is directly related to the time taken for a patient to reach a definitive surgical treatment.

Box 1.3 Larrey and Percy: The Beginnings of a Systematic Approach to Trauma Management

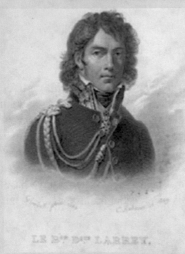 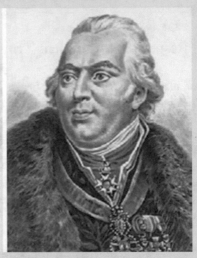

LE B.^T DR LARREY.

Source Wikimedia Commons.
http://commons.wikimedia.org/wiki/File:Dominique_Jean_Larrey_-_engraving.jpg.
http://commons.wikimedia.org/wiki/File:PierreFrancoisPercy.jpg.

Baron Larrey is familiar to many English-speaking doctors for his groundbreaking contributions to triage and the rapid evacuation of the wounded from the battlefield. His contemporary and compatriot Pierre-François Percy (whose name is immortalised to this day in the newest of the Parisian military hospitals) is less familiar outside France, but his contribution to casualty management was no less than that of Larrey.

Dominique Jean Larrey was born near Bagnères de Bigorre in the Pyrénées on 6 July 1766. Orphaned at the age of nine he followed the career of his uncle, a surgeon at Toulouse. After studying in Lyon, he went to Paris in 1786 shortly before the French Revolution with the intention of continuing his surgical studies, but instead he joined the Royal French Navy. He did not remain in the navy (he suffered from chronic seasickness) but returned instead to continue his studies at the Hôtel-Dieu hospital, beside the cathedral of Notre Dame in Paris.

In 1792, he joined the Army of the Rhine as an assistant surgeon and served in Corsica and Spain before becoming professor of surgery at the great military hospital of Val de Grace in Paris. The French Army was becoming reformed and highly effective under the leadership of the 26-year-old General Bonaparte with whom Larrey soon became a favourite. Larrey accompanied him on his campaigns to Egypt, Palestine and Syria and undertook a complete reorganisation of the field medical services which hitherto had been rudimentary in common with other armies at that time. Larrey was appointed surgeon-in-chief to the French Army in 1805 and took part in increasingly bloody campaigns in Germany and Poland as well as the ill-fated expedition to Russia in 1812. Larrey's busy medical life was to continue for another 27 years. After the restoration, he was appointed inspector general of the Medical Service and held surgical posts at the Garde Royale and the Hôpital des Invalides in Paris as well as organising the medical service of the newly created Belgian Republic in 1831.

Pierre-François Percy (1754–1825) was born at Montagney in Haute Saône on 28 October 1754 a decade before Larrey. His active military career was to span three decades: first in the service of Louis XVI and then for Napoleon, where, as inspector general of the Medical Service, he introduced a major reorganisation. Percy was surgeon to the Grande Armée in 1803 at the time of the aborted invasion of England. Percy took part in some of the bloodiest battles of the wars including Austerlitz (1805), Jena (1806), Eylau (1807), Wagram (1809) and the Spanish campaign of 1808–1809. After the battle of Eylau, Percy wrote graphically of the plight of the wounded for whom there was practically no organisation, a fact which came to the attention of Napoleon who ordered radical changes in the provision of surgical care. After Wagram, Percy, because of his age and health, withdrew from active campaigning and devoted his time to administration of the army health services and to teaching at the University of Paris. He was, however, created a member of the newly formed Academy of Medicine in 1820.

It was realised after the Vietnam War that early life-support interventions after injury were critical to clinical outcome, and the American traumatologist R. Adams Cowley introduced the concept of the 'Golden Hour' to emphasise this fact. Deaths following physical trauma come in three distinct waves. The first comprises persons who die within 30 min as a result of complex and overwhelming injury from which survival is impossible, such as major brain or vascular damage. The second wave, which comprises 30 % of the injuries, occurs after about 4 h and is the result of a combination of blood loss leading to shock and cellular damage and failure to maintain an adequate airway and ventilation. Airway obstruction, in particular, has been estimated to contribute to the death of 40 % of the victims.

The third peak which comprises 20 % of all physical trauma deaths represents patients who die within days or weeks of injury as a result of long-term complications. It has long been recognised that physical trauma can have longer-term complications and consequences. Infection and gangrene were common and life threatening well into the twentieth century. More recently, the longer-term consequences of trauma have been recognised by the effects on the various organ systems of the body. In many cases, physical trauma can lead to serious complications such as the acute respiratory distress syndrome (ARDS) and multiple organ failure which require treatment in intensive care units. But the growth of intensive care medicine itself and improved surgical techniques has changed the prognostic outcome for trauma and has fuelled research into a better understanding of the mechanisms involved.

The overall message from the development of the management of physical trauma is that an early and systematic intervention which addresses not only the immediate trauma but also the maintenance of life support in the form of airway, breathing and circulation can have a dramatic effect on the outcome. This approach has much relevance to the management of injury from toxic chemical agents.

1.4   Toxic Trauma

During the early part of the twentieth century, it became apparent that serious injury to the body can occur not only as a result of physical trauma but also from exposure to toxic chemical substances. A toxic substance is conventionally defined as an extraneous chemical substance, which has the ability to cause harm to living organisms both directly and indirectly. The concept of a poisonous substance has been understood for many thousands of years, but it was during the sixteenth century and later that the nature of poisons was defined by alchemists and physicians such as Paracelsus and Matteo Orfila (see Chap. 3), which led to the beginning of the science of toxicology. Individual poisoning is most familiar through its effects by ingestion, whether accidental or deliberate. However, following the development of the chemical industry during the nineteenth century, it was quickly realised that many chemical substances have the ability to cause harm to the body as a result of direct exposure and entry from routes other than ingestion, notably through inhalation, and which can cause damage to a number of somatic systems. As a result, the concept of damage to the body from toxic chemicals perhaps requires a broader definition than 'poisoning'.

We have seen that trauma to the body can be produced from a variety of causes which form part of a spectrum which includes penetrating, and blunt trauma and also thermal trauma from burns and cold injury. These various forms of injury can have both immediate and long-term effects, and there are common terminal pathways of cell and organ damage and death.

The actions of toxic chemicals on the body can be integrated into the various forms of physical trauma by using the concept of 'toxic trauma'.

Toxic trauma can be defined broadly as the disruption of somatic systems and their function by exposure to a toxic chemical. Ingested poisoning in its conventional form is only one example of toxic trauma. As we shall see in later chapters, toxic exposure can also arise from inhalation of gases or exposure of the skin to liquids or solids. Like physical trauma, toxic trauma can produce early or late effects with potential fatality at all stages.

The integration of physical and toxic trauma has a number of advantages. Firstly, it highlights common initial problems such as hypoxia and shock and, later, life-threatening complications. An example is found in ARDS which can follow both blast injury to the lung and inhalation of lung-damaging agents such as chlorine. Although the relationship between toxic trauma and blunt and penetrating physical trauma may not be immediately obvious, the similarities with thermal trauma (both hot and cold) and the actions of corrosive substances such as acids and alkalis are more familiar. Importantly, both physical and toxic trauma may lead to a common management within the intensive care unit in extreme cases. Both may cause a severe strain on medical resources in the case of mass injury which is increasingly a feature of modern civil life as a result of terrorist action. Secondly, an integrated approach to trauma emphasises the importance of an early and systematic approach to emergency care.

1.5   The Epidemiology of Toxic Trauma

The deliberate release of chemicals to produce toxic trauma has been familiar in warfare for more than 2000 years. In civil life, although there may have been coincidental exposure (e.g. in siege warfare), most acute toxic trauma up to the twentieth century would have been due to ingested poisonous substances. Since that time, civilians have been increasingly at risk from exposure to both agents of chemical warfare and toxic industrial chemicals.

The emergence of terrorist use of chemicals over the past two decades, as well as the increasing risk of exposure to accidental release of toxic industrial chemicals, makes the appearance in hospital of casualties with toxic trauma more likely. Emergency medical teams may have to respond quickly to an unfamiliar situation, particularly since the abolition of military service in many countries has produced a generation of civilian doctors and nurses who do not have direct experience of planning and management of such situations as was the case following the two world wars.

Despite attempts in the late nineteenth century to ban the use of chemicals in warfare (the Hague convention of 1899 failed because it related only to the use of chemicals in projectiles), chemical warfare was used extensively during World War I and produced casualties who were recognisably suffering from toxic rather than physical trauma. Some had both. It was the use of chemicals in warfare and the multiple short- and long-term effects on body systems that pointed the way to the need to approach trauma from exposure to chemicals in the same systematic way as for physical trauma.

In everyday life, there is an increasing risk of accidental and deliberate mass exposure to toxic chemical agents causing acute and potentially life-threatening effects as well as chronic effects lasting many years. Examples of mass chemical injury in the civil setting include the Bhopal disaster in 1984 where the accidental release of methyl isocyanate from a chemical plant in India caused the death of several thousands of people and chronically injured over 50,000 more (see Chap. 10). In the military setting, chemical agents remain a potent threat and have been used within living memory in the Iran–Iraq War during the 1980s and during the Syrian Civil War.

As has been noted, toxic trauma occurs in both the military setting, where the release of chemicals specifically designed to cause harm is a deliberate action or in civil life, where the release is usually accidental and involves toxic industrial chemicals that are used in chemical engineering and have coincidental harmful effects. The continued development, transport and use of toxic industrial chemicals and the increasing likelihood of accidental and deliberate release make toxic trauma in civilians and their need for pre-hospital and hospital treatment an increasingly likely occurrence.

With the steady growth of the production, transport and use of toxic chemicals around the world, there has been an increase in the number of casualties with toxic trauma. Although the end of the Cold War reduced the risk of major chemical attacks, the stockpiles of chemical weapons remained and may have fallen into the hands of terrorists. The release of the nerve agent sarin in the Tokyo metro in 1995 confirmed the ability of terrorist organisations not only to use chemical weapons but also to synthesise them. In summary, mass exposure to toxic substances remains a relatively rare but significant event which has importance for emergency medicine and several other specialities.

1.6   The Clinical Importance of Toxic Trauma

Acute toxic exposure is part of the disciplines of both emergency medicine and clinical toxicology. For most emergency physicians, acute exposure means accidental or self-poisoning through the ingestion route. Individual poisoning is familiar in the hospital setting in both the developed and the developing world. Exposure to toxic substances has particular importance for emergency medical responders who themselves may be at risk of injury whilst caring for the casualties following the toxic release. Toxic exposure covers a wider setting than individual ingestion poisoning which is familiar within the emergency department.

Toxic chemical agents injure through a variety of routes of entry into the body and by affecting several somatic systems. An understanding of the pathophysiogical process involved is essential to management. Mass physical trauma is increasingly familiar to doctors and surgeons working in both the military and the civil settings as a result of continuing wars and civil terrorist activity. However, exposure to toxic substances either individually or *en masse* is by comparison a relatively unusual event, and it is important that emergency medical teams are as familiar with the injuries caused as they are with conventional physical trauma. This means not only the effective early and continuing clinical management of victims but also the awareness of the dangers to responders of secondary injury and knowledge in how to counter these.

1.7   Approaches to Trauma Management

A systematic approach to the management of physical trauma is now common worldwide. The management of trauma caused by chemical substances has not received the same attention although an approach following the ATLS^{TM} model to the management of exposure to hazardous materials has also been developed with the US Advanced Hazmat Life Support (AHLS) course (Box 1.4). However, toxic injury is still largely regarded as being separate from physical injury and does not always receive sufficiently detailed holistic medical approach as part of a spectrum of mechanisms and management of trauma. The reasons for this may be due to the relative infrequency of toxic trauma (as opposed to conventional poisoning) in pre-hospital and hospital emergency medicine.

Box 1.4 Advanced Hazmat Life-Support Course
Following the precedent set in the management of physical trauma by the ATLS training, the AHLS courses teach healthcare professionals to medically manage patients exposed to hazardous materials, including chemical, biological and radiological incidents.

This course covers hazardous materials including pesticides, corrosives, irritant gases, asphyxiants, hydrocarbons and halogenated hydrocarbons and chemical, biological, radiological and nuclear agents. Specific antidotes and their indications, contraindications, dosing and route are also included.

Source http://www.ahls.org.ahls/ees/main/ahls_home.html. Accessed 21 July 2013

1.8   Conclusion

This chapter has introduced a concept of toxic trauma which forms part of a wider spectrum of physical trauma in its many forms. This approach has the advantages of integrating the understanding and management of injury from exposure to toxic substances into emergency and continuing medical management. For emergency physicians whose experience of toxic trauma is largely confined to the management of ingested poisons, this integrated approach may be helpful in management, particularly of mass toxic casualties. The subsequent chapters of this book will consider the nature and classification of toxic hazards, both military and civil, and how people can suffer acute exposure to them from accidental or deliberate release. Then, the pathophysiology of toxic trauma is discussed and its clinical presentation and management with particular emphasis on the application of life-support measures. Although this book is concerned essentially with the acute presentation of toxic trauma, there is a section on the longer-term consequences where continuing hospital management is required. Finally, we consider examples of large-scale release of toxic chemical agents in both war and peace and the lessons they illustrate for emergency medical responders.

Further Reading

Advanced Trauma Life Support (2016) http://www.facs.org/trauma/atls/history.atm/. Accessed 21 July 2013
Advanced Hazmat Life Support (2016) http://www.ahls.org.ahls/ecs/main/ahls_home.html. Accessed 21 July 2013
Shamir MY, Weiss YG (eds) (2007) Trauma. Anesthesiol Clin 25(1) (WB Saunders, Philadelphia)
Trunkey DD (1983) Trauma. Sci Am 249:20–27
Urbanetti J, Newmark J (2010) Clinical aspects of large scale chemical events. In: Koenig KL, Schultz CH (eds) Disaster medicine: comprehensive principles and practices. Cambridge University Press, New York

Chapter 2
Toxic Trauma: A Historical Perspective

Abstract Exposure to toxic chemicals goes back at least 2000 years with the first use of irritating agents such as smokes and burning sulphur in warfare, a practice which continued until the Middle Ages. The industrial revolution and the development of large-scale chemical industries in Europe laid the basis for the large-scale chemical warfare seen in the First World War. Throughout the remainder of the twentieth century and beyond there were continuing occurrences of mass exposure to chemicals, not only from deliberate release in chemical warfare but also from accidental release by an ever-expanding chemical industry. These had particularly severe consequences in developing countries with limited emergency responses. This chapter presents a brief historical perspective of the toxic trauma produced from exposure to chemical substances in both the military and civil settings.

2.1 Exposure to Chemicals From Early Times to the Nineteenth Century

Man has learned the dangers of poisonous substances in the wild since his days as a hunter-gatherer in pre-history. Exposure to toxic agents in warfare and in peace also dates back many thousands of years. As long ago as 2000 BC, toxic smokes were being used in battle in China and India. They are also recorded by Thucydides in around 500 BC. The Athenian general described the first use of chemicals in

© Springer International Publishing Switzerland 2016
D.J. Baker, *Toxic Trauma*, DOI 10.1007/978-3-319-40916-0_2

Western warfare in his history of the Peloponnesian War, which took place between 431 and 404 BC. (Box 2.1) The Romans also, around 80 BC, used a toxic smoke in battles which caused blindness and choking pulmonary symptoms.

Box 2.1 Thucydides and the First Use of Chemical Warfare

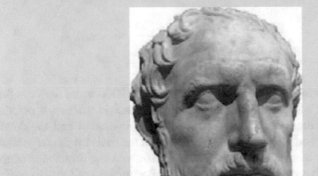

Source Wikimedia Commons http://commons.wikimedia.org/wiki/File:Paracelsus.jpg

The Athenian general and historian Thucydides (c. 460–c. 395 BC) described the first use of chemical warfare in Western civilisation, by Sparta against Athens, in his *History of the Peloponnesian War* (431-404 BC). Wood was saturated with pitch and sulphur and then burned under the walls of the city during the siege of Plataea in 428 BC to produce poisonous choking fumes (as well as fear and panic). The use of fire and poisonous fumes continued to be a weapon of siege warfare until well beyond the Middle Ages.

The concept of an incendiary chemical device was developed by Callinus in Constantinople around 670 AD with the development and use of Greek Fire. This was an autocombustive mixture of resin, pitch sulphur, naphtha, quicklime and saltpetre (later to be a main constituent of gunpowder). The mixture ignited on contact with water and burned on the surface of the sea, causing immense damage to enemy vessels. Incendiary devices which produced toxic fumes continued to be used through the Middle Ages and Renaissance.

Agents that caused pulmonary toxic trauma (see Chap. 6) were being used and considered in the Middle Ages following the use of fire and smoke in earlier sieges. Leonardo da Vinci himself proposed the use of a mixture of sulphur, arsenic and copper acetate as a lung-damaging warfare agent. In 1672, Christoph Bernhard von Galen, the Bishop of Munster, used a number of incendiary devices designed to produce toxic fumes. This led to the 1675 Strasbourg agreement which represented the first attempt to control the use of toxic substances in warfare, a process which has continued to the present day.

2.2   The Industrial Revolution and the Development of Mass Chemical Warfare

The foundations of modern chemical warfare (CW) agents in the twentieth century were made possible by the creation of large industrial chemical facilities in Europe in the nineteenth century. The astonishing range of chemicals that were tested and used as CW agents during World War I was made possible by the industrial revolution and particularly by the chance discovery of aniline dyes by the British chemist William Perkin (Box 2.2) in the mid-nineteenth century. Perkin built up a major British synthetic dye industry which was then overtaken by a number of German companies. This opened the pathway to the creation of industrial chemical giants such as IG Farben which allowed the mass production and stockpiling of chemical agents at the beginning of World War I and the development of new chemical agents between the wars.

Box 2.2 William Perkin: The Father of Modern Synthetic Dyes

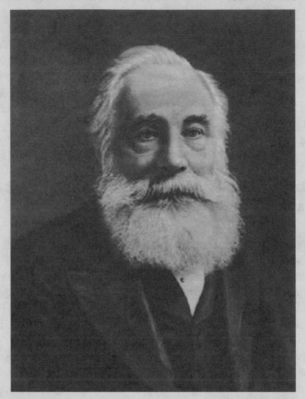

Source Wikimedia Commons http://commons.wikimedia.org/wiki/File:William_Perkin.jpg

William Perkin was born in the East End of London, the youngest of the seven children of George Perkin, a successful carpenter. In 1853, at the age of only 15, Perkin entered the Royal College of Chemistry in London (now part of Imperial College London), where he began his studies under the distinguished German chemist August Wilhelm von Hofmann. Although he was working on the chemistry of quinine, Perkin performed his own experiments in the crude laboratory in his apartment on the top floor of his home in East London. It was here that he made the discovery that aniline could be partly transformed to produce a substance with an intense purple colour which he called Mauveine. Perkin's discovery came at a time when the industrial revolution had created major improvements in the production of textiles. Chemistry now had a major impact on industrial processes, and coal tar, the major source of Perkin's raw material, was an abundant by-product of the process for making coal gas and coke. Perkin set up a successful factory that was to become the basis of the synthetic dye industry in the UK. The technology spread to Germany, a country that was to become dominant in the field by the end of the nineteenth century, leading to the establishment of a chemical industry that would provide the basis for the production of chemical warfare agents.

2.3 First Suggested Uses of Chemical Weapons in the Nineteenth Century

The first suggested military use of chemicals as weapons took place in the middle of the nineteenth century when the British chemist Lyon Playfair proposed in 1854, the use of a cyanide shell to break the siege at Sevastopol in the Crimea. Nearly a decade later, in the American Civil War, John Doughty suggested the use of a chorine shell against an entrenched enemy. Neither of these suggestions was adopted, but full-scale CW was to become a stark reality 50 years later in the First World War when extensive use of toxic agents was made by both sides, starting with the use of chlorine by the German in April 1915. There was growing awareness of the threat of CW towards the end of the century, and the 1899 Hague Convention banned the use of chemical agents in warfare, but only if delivered by shell or other projectiles.

2.4 The First World War

The First World War saw the beginning of mass use of toxic chemical agents in battle. This has been exhaustively analysed by military historians and is the subject of a number of detailed texts, some of which are listed at the end of this chapter. At the time of writing, the first gas attack occurred 100 years ago and the detailed experience of the emergency medical and nursing personnel who had to deal with casualties of this new form of warfare has been largely forgotten. However, the war provides many valuable lessons for modern emergency responders in the management of toxic trauma which are still relevant.

The chemical attacks of the first war could not have taken place without the backing of the German chemical industry and the scientists working within it. The original use of the chlorine and phosgene in 1915 was coordinated by the chemist Fritz Haber who is best known for his chemical synthesis of ammonia to produce explosives, for which he received the Nobel Prize for chemistry in 1919. Haber directed the enormous resources of the German chemical industry, originally based on the production of dyestuffs into mass production of CW agents (Box 2.3). Use of chemical weapons, although banned by the Hague Convention, was rapidly adopted by both sides and caused many millions of casualties.

Box 2.3 Fritz Haber

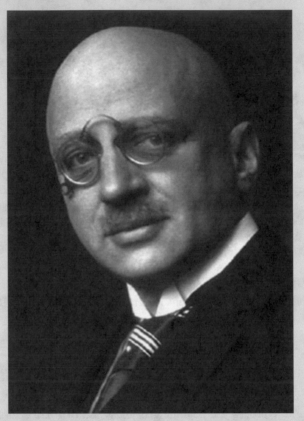

Source Wikimedia Commons http://commons.wikimedia.org/wiki/File:Fritz_Haber.png

Fritz Haber (1934) was a German chemist and professor at the Kaiser Wilhelm Institute in Berlin who received the Nobel Prize in 1919 for his innovative work on the production of synthetic nitrates from ammonia. This was in fact driven by the need for their requirements in the production of explosives in the First World War after the blockade of raw materials from Chile. Haber worked in the IG Farben group of companies, initially set up as the name suggests for the production of dyes but whose chemical engineering expertise was diverted to the production of chemical warfare agents. IG Farben (*Interessen Gemeinschaft Farben,* literally, community of interests, of dye-making corporation) was a union of six German chemical companies who dominated the synthetic dye industry before the First World War. In 1913, Germany produced over 85 % of the world's dyes (the UK by this stage only produced 2.5 % and the USA 2 %). Haber was closely associated with the planning of the first major gas attack at Ypres in 1915 where chlorine was released from cylinders (thus not violating the Hague Convention of

1899 which only prohibited the use of toxic gases in artillery shells) but was said to be frustrated by the failure of the military to follow through the successful attack and end the war. Chlorine was selected by Haber because it was lethal, had a short latency of action and was non-persistent. It could form a dense toxic cloud able to resist dilution in a moderate wind but with no prolonged effect on the terrain. Haber was also associated with the development of phosgene and sulphur mustard gas, first used in July 1917, again at Ypres. Haber was Jewish and was forced out of Germany in 1934 after the rise of the Nazis. He died in Switzerland shortly afterwards.

Early experimental attacks by both sides using irritant (tear gas) agents had taken place in late 1914 and early 1915 on both the western and eastern fronts with mixed results. However, this signalled the way to disregard the Hague Convention and to launch attacks with potentially lethal CW agents.

The first major chemical attack took place at Ypres in Belgium on 22 April 1915. The German Army released 168 tons of chlorine gas from nearly 6000 cylinders (which were not covered by the Hague Convention) on to the French lines with devastating results. Although the accurate figure is not known, the number of French and North African troops killed in the attack is thought to have been around 10,000. The attack produced a gap of nearly 9 miles on the western front, but the German commander, von Falkenhayn, did not believe the reports he had heard about this; he had no reserves available to exploit the advantage, complete the German assault on to Paris and thus end the war. Within 2 days, British and Canadian troops had secured the line and the military advantage had been lost. Only one subsequent attack, at Bolimov on the eastern front where the Germans attacked Russian troops, was to have such a devastating effect. This time, 262 tons of chlorine was released from 12,000 cylinders along a line of 7.5 miles producing 25,000 casualties and 6000 dead. This was a lesson about CW the Russians never forgot up to and beyond the Second World War.

Countermeasures to the initial attacks were quickly introduced, including primitive gas masks and better training, and the catastrophic effects of the first gas attacks were never repeated. Nevertheless, in combination with other arms, toxic chemicals proved to be a continuing and influential factor in the largely static warfare of the first war.

Chlorine was quickly replaced by the Germans with diphosgene and phosgene (first used in December 1915). Phosgene, with its early upper respiratory irritant effects and late onset pulmonary oedema (see Chap. 6), proved to be one of the most dangerous agents of the war.

Inhaled gas warfare continued to be a major factor in the trench warfare of 1916, but in 1917, a new agent, sulphur mustard gas, was used by the Germans with continuing success. Mustard gas was designed to disable combatants rather than to kill, and it proved to be one of the most insidious of CW agents. It still remains a major military and terrorist threat up to the present day.

More than 60 chemical compounds were tested during World War I, but only a few found extensive use as chemical weapons. The most notable were chlorine, phosgene, hydrogen cyanide, arsines and mustard gas. The vesicant Lewisite which had quicker actions than mustard gas was produced in 1919 and not used during the war. Of these compounds, it is noteworthy that three of them are toxic industrial chemicals (TIC) and are still being produced in large quantities by the chemical industry today.

Despite the ban on the use of chemical projectiles which was in force in 1914, by the end of the war, chemical shells were widely used. Had the war continued into 1919, it was predicted that more than half of the shell fills would have been chemical.

Despite their mass disabling actions, CW agents produced the lowest dead-to-wounded ratio of all the weapons used in World War I (4 % as opposed to over 12 % from artillery). The high proportion of the latter reflects the limited responses to major physical trauma at the time. By the end of the twentieth century and after the application of advanced life-support measures in battle for physical and toxic trauma, both ratios have steadily decreased.

2.5   Between the World Wars

The Geneva chemical weapons convention of 1925 banned the first use but not the stockpiling of chemical weapons. Most countries ratified the treaty quickly but the USA did not do so until 1975. There are still three countries, North Korea, Syria and Israel, who still have not ratified the treaty at the time of writing.

Despite the indignant reaction against chemical weapons during and after the First World War, most combatant countries had learned lessons from the new warfare and proceeded with development and training. The Russians in particular who had suffered over 400,000 wounded and 56,000 dead were quick to build up their chemical capability, ironically under the guidance of ex-officers of the former Imperial German Army. Russian chemical capability continued with the formation of special chemical battalions in the Second World War that were not involved in general fighting duties, even during the battle of Stalingrad. The lessons of the first war were not forgotten.

2.5.1   The 1930s: First Systematic Use of Chemical Warfare Agents Against Civil Populations

Despite the 1925 treaty, the following decade saw the continued production and use of CW agents against civil populations.

In 1936, the Italian Army used mustard gas against a poorly trained and equipped army and civilians in Abyssinia as part of a systematic campaign of CW. Waves of aircraft drenched combatants and civilians and polluted rivers, lakes and pastures. The devastating effects of this campaign, which caused tens of thousands of victims, were a major contribution to the Italian victory and the occupation of Abyssinia until the British liberation during World War II.

The wider effect of this campaign was to alert nations that were about to fight World War II of the effects of aerial gas attacks against a civilian population. As a result, by 1939, there was mass production of gas masks in the UK and Germany. In the event, gas was not used by either side in Europe during World War I, but the threat was always regarded as high.

Elsewhere, during the Manchurian War between Japan and China which started in 1937 and which some historians regard as effectively the beginning of World War II in the Far East, chemical weapons, notably mustard gas, were used against civilian populations in a number of attacks. At that time, Japan had not ratified the 1925 Geneva CW treaty. By 1941, there were reports that there had been over 800 attacks against the Chinese Nationalists of Chiang Kai-shek using mainly mustard gas. There were continuing fears in the USA that the Japanese would use gas weapons against them, but in the event, the Japanese wound down their CW training and production ability as the war progressed against them, possibly for fear of reprisals.

2.6   The Second World War

Despite the growing fears in the 1930s, chemical weapons were not used in Europe during the Second World War either in battle or against civilians. Historians debate the reasons for this, but one major factor affecting German use was their diminishing air capability as the war progressed and the fear of aerial reprisals by the Allies with their overwhelming air superiority by 1945.

The nonuse of CW agents, however, did not stop the production and stockpiling of chemical weapons. In one of the worst mustard gas releases recorded, more than a thousand sailors and civilians were killed on 2 December 1943 in Bari harbour in Italy. In one of the heaviest raids of the war, more than 100 German JU88 bombers attacked packed Allied shipping in the harbour, producing the most devastating attack of its type since Pearl Harbour. Seventeen ships carrying over 90,000 tons of supplies were sunk. One of the ships moored in the harbour, the John Harvey, was carrying a cargo of mustard gas bombs. As the ship sank, liquid mustard gas was released onto the surface of the water where it combined with floating oil. Hundreds of sailors in the water who had abandoned the ship suffered heavy contamination. The result of the attack was a mass influx of mustard casualties into hospitals who had no idea of the cause of the wounds, which because of the very heavy contamination were severe and lead to early deaths.

The Bari disaster influenced opinion anew about the disastrous consequences of mass CW and possibly was the first event to lead to CW agents being considered as weapons of 'mass destruction'.

2.6.1   The Secret Development of Nerve Agents

In 1936, Gerhardt Schrader (Box 2.4) who also worked for IG Farben in Germany discovered the first nerve gas (tabun) as an offshoot of research into organophosphate pesticide compounds. The nerve gases (considered in detail in subsequent chapters) were the most toxic substances discovered. Schrader's work was reported to the German High Command and was immediately given the highest security classification. As a result, the Allies were unaware of the research and production that had taken place even by the time of victory in 1945. Schrader and his colleagues Ambros, Rudiger and van der Linde went on to synthesise the other nerve agents, sarin and soman. Sarin derives its name from an acronym of the researchers. By 1945, the Germans have produced about 12,000 tons of tabun and about 1000 tons of sarin. The capture of the production plant at Dyhernfurth in Poland by the Russians and its subsequent shipping to Volgograd where it was reconstructed saw the beginning of the Cold War chemical arms race that was to last for more than 40 years.

Box 2.4 Gerhardt Schrader

Gerhard Schrader (25 February 1903–1990) was a German chemist specialising in the discovery of new insecticides, Schrader is best known for his accidental discovery of nerve agents such as sarin and tabun. In 1936, while employed by the large German conglomerate IG Farben (who later supplied Zyklon B, a hydrogen cyanide compound for use in the Nazi extermination camps), he was experimenting with organophosphate compounds (known at that time for nearly 80 years) as insecticides. Schrader discovered several very effective insecticides, including bladan (the first fully synthetic contact insecticide) and parathion. While searching for a new insecticide, he accidentally discovered tabun, the first chemical warfare nerve agent and later sarin (a name formed from the initials of Schrader and his collaborators). Schrader's discovery was placed under the tightest secrecy by the Nazis, and he continued to work on the development of further nerve agents during the Second World War. Nerve agents were not used in that war and their development was not detected by Allied intelligence services until the defeat of Germany in 1945. The plant producing sarin was captured by the Red Army and transported to Volgograd in the USSR where it continued production and started the chemical arms race of the Cold War.

2.7   The Cold War Period

Following the end of the Second World War, the Allied powers established secret research and production facilities based on the German work on nerve agents. Academic research into the effects of these and new compounds was supported by special contracts in the USA and by the creation of special state research institutes in the Union of Soviet Socialist Republics (USSR). Open publications during the period reported toxicological studies on both animals and human volunteers. Training for protection against CW agents became a feature of all sides during the Cold War with the development of new treatment measures and antidotes.

A large number of publications indicated that there was considerable interest in toxins (see Chap. 11) and the development of new chemical compounds such as short-chain neuropeptides which could affect thinking and consciousness and severely affect fighting ability. Toxins, although chemical in nature, are produced by biological organisms and are not classed as CW agents. Their use would not therefore violate the 1925 Geneva treaty.

2.8   Continued Military Use of Chemical Warfare Agents

Despite the treaty obligations, CW agents were used in a number of wars after 1945 although the facts in many cases are often hard to establish due to the intense secrecy that surrounded and still surrounds the subject.

There was alleged use of chemical agents including nerve agents and mustard gas in Yemen between 1963 and 1967 and also of trichothecene toxins in Cambodia during the Vietnam War. However, the most extensive use of both nerve and mustard agents took place during the Iran–Iraq war in the 1980s where the Iranians suffered over 20,000 casualties from the use of nerve agents and mustard gas. This was the first war where chemical casualties were assessed and managed using modern medical techniques with a consequent reduction in the number of fatalities from that seen in the First World War.

In 1995, there was the first documented use of a CW agent by terrorists in a civil setting with the release of sarin in the Japanese cities of Matsumoto and Tokyo. These incidents again raised public awareness of the vulnerability of unprotected civil populations to toxic agents. These incidents are discussed in more detail in Chap. 10.

2.9 Mass Accidental Release of Toxic Industrial Chemicals

The increasing use and transportation of toxic industrial chemicals around the world following the Second World War has been accompanied by a rise in the number of small- and large-scale accidental releases causing toxic trauma in the civil setting. The most devastating of this was in Bhopal in India in 1984 where the accidental release of 40 tons of methyl isocyanate, a chemical intermediary in the production of pesticide and other compounds in a densely populated urban area, led to more than 5000 fatalities. The important medical lessons from this incident are considered in Chap. 10.

2.10 Conclusions

The deliberate release of toxic chemicals has been a feature of warfare for more than 2000 years. Up to the age of enlightenment, it was conducted on only a small scale, but the arrival of the industrial revolution saw the creation of a civil chemical industry that could support the mass production and use of chemical agents in warfare. The First World War caused mass casualties and fatalities from this form of warfare, which had been described as the most significant development in arms since the invention of gunpowder. Since that time, CW agents have been used on a regular basis and have proved to be particularly effective against unprotected civilian populations. In addition, deliberate release of chemical agents has now been proven to be within the capability of terrorist organisations. Accidental release of toxic industrial chemicals has been an increasing feature of the twentieth century and beyond. An understanding of the basic history of the development and use of chemical agents and lessons from accidental release is more than valuable for a structured approach towards effective management of toxic trauma, considered in the following chapters. Box 2.5 gives a timeline of the history of chemical releases, both deliberate and accidental over the past 100 years.

> **Box 2.5 One hundred years of toxic trauma: a timeline of events**
> 1915 January: First use of tear gas shells on the Russian front in Poland
>   April: First recorded chemical warfare attack at Ypres, Belgium, using chlorine gas released from cylinders. Over 10,000 dead from inhalation of high concentrations of gas
>   May: Chlorine used at the Battle of Bolimov on the eastern front. Six thousand Russian soldiers killed with 25,000 further casualties
>   December: Phosgene used against the British at Ypres
>   1916: Continued effective use of phosgene and also attacks using hydrogen cyanide
>   1917 July: First use of mustard gas at Ypres. Four thousand British casualties of whom 500 died within 3 weeks

1919: Development of the rapid-acting vesicant Lewisite (never used in battle)

1936: Use of mustard gas in the Italian Ethiopian campaign

1936–1945: Discovery and production of nerve gases in Germany

1938–1941: Probable use of mustard gas and other chemical agents in the Sino–Japanese Manchurian war

1943: Explosion of US liberty ship carrying mustard gas shells in Bari harbour, Italy

1945: Beginning of the Cold War chemical arms race

1968: Probable use of mycotoxin agents in the Vietnam War

1963–1967: Use of nerve and mustard agents in the Yemen

1984: Bhopal, India. Release of 40 tons of methyl isocyanate into an urban residential area. More than 5000 deaths and more than 50,000 injured, many with long-term lung problems

1984–1988: Use of nerve agents and mustard gas in the Iran–Iraq War. Substantial casualties but a reduced mortality due to overall improvements in medical care

1988: Use of nerve and mustard agents on a civil population in Halabja, Kurdistan. More than 5000 fatalities

1975–1992: Development of a new generation of powerful nerve agents (Novichocks) by the USSR

1994–1995: First substantiated use of a chemical weapon (sarin nerve gas) by a terrorist organisation in a civil setting. Matsumoto and Tokyo, Japan

2002: Use of a calmative 'knockdown' agent by Russian special forces during the Moscow theatre siege. More than 160 fatalities

2006: Chlorine improvised explosive device used in Iraq

2013–2015: Use of CW agents (sarin, sulphur mustard and chlorine) against civilians during the Syrian Civil War

Further Reading

Alibek K (2000) Biohazard. Arrow Books, London, UK

Hill BA (2008) History of the medical management of chemical casualties. In: Tuorinsky SD (ed) Medical aspects of chemical warfare office of the surgeon general, US Army. Borden Institute, Washington DC, pp 77–114 (Chap. 3)

Hilmas CJ, Smart JK, Hill BA (2008) History of chemical warfare. In: Tuorinsky SD (ed) Medical aspects of chemical warfare office of the surgeon general, US Army. Borden Institute, Washington, pp 9–76 (Chap. 2)

Paxman J, Harris R (2002) A higher form of killing: the secret history of chemical and biological warfare. Arrow Books, London

Prentiss AM (1937) Chemicals in war: a treatise on chemical warfare. McGraw—Hill Inc, New York

Tucker JB (2007) War of nerves: chemical warfare from World war 1 to Al-Queda. Anchor Books, New York

Chapter 3
The Classification and Properties of Toxic Hazards

Abstract A wide range of toxic hazards exist, both natural and man-made. A toxic hazard may be defined as any substance which has the ability to cause harm or damage to living organisms. The term 'toxin' is often used synonymously with any poison, but should be reserved to mean any toxic chemical which originates from a biological organism. Toxic trauma is the result of acute exposure to hazardous substances that cause life-threatening, seriously disabling acute effects and the intermediate effects that follow. Toxic agents may be classed as toxic industrial chemicals (TIC) or agents of chemical warfare (CW). Some agents such as chlorine and phosgene are both TIC and CW agents. Both TIC and CW agents may be classified in terms of their actions on somatic systems. TIC are also classified and identified using the UN HAZMAT system which assigns each agent into one of nine classes and gives an identification code number. Each toxic agent has four distinct properties, physical form, persistency toxicity and latency, which determine their action in the body and also the risks of transmission of the hazard to other persons.

3.1 Introduction

There exist a wide range of toxic hazards which are both natural and man-made. These may affect humans both individually and collectively, producing mass casualties. The potential hazards to which humans may be exposed are different in different parts of the world. These depend on such factors as industrialisation, availability of chemical substances for everyday domestic and industrial use, waste-handling procedures, flora and fauna. In the wider sense, mass toxic exposure and the vulnerability of unprotected populations to deliberate chemical release must be considered together with such factors as terrorism and the local stockpiling of chemical warfare (CW) agents. This chapter considers the classification and properties of toxic chemical agents, whether CW agents or toxic industrial chemicals (TIC) and their physical and biological properties.

© Springer International Publishing Switzerland 2016
D.J. Baker, *Toxic Trauma*, DOI 10.1007/978-3-319-40916-0_3

3.2   Toxic Hazards: Definitions

A toxic hazard may be defined as any substance which has the ability to cause harm or damage to living organisms. Until the last century, the acute effects of toxic agent were most familiar as ingested poisons. Poisons have been known since early times, with most sources being plants. In addition, the effects of envenomation from snakes and insects have also been recognised. About 500 years ago, there was the beginning of a wider understanding of the nature of poisons, led by Paracelsus who recognised that all substances were potentially poisonous, and not just a few recognised substances. The determining factor was the dose. Following the industrial revolution and the development of chemistry and the chemical industry, the number of recognised poisonous substances increased dramatically, and there was an understanding that they could enter the body by routes other than ingestion or envenomation.

As noted previously, the term 'toxic agent' means any substance causing toxic trauma. This includes conventional poisons such as cyanide and arsenic but also includes any substance which can cause harm to body systems acutely. The term 'toxin' is often used synonymously with any poison but should be reserved to mean any toxic agent which has a biological origin. Examples are bacterial and animal toxins. Although from biological origin, these are essentially chemical in nature. Many of these have been extracted and produced in large quantities for possible use as agents of CW and therefore are a potential cause of mass toxic trauma. Toxins have been excluded from treaties that control agents of CW and are considered to be agents of biological warfare. However, their actions in the body fall within the definition of toxic trauma. Toxins therefore form an important subclass of chemical agents. More details about their nature and actions are presented in Chap. 11.

3.3   Acute and Chronic Toxic Hazards

The standard definition of a toxic agent includes substances that cause both acute and latent effects with both short and long duration. Chronic exposure to low doses of toxic agents has been increasingly recognised as a cause of illness and is the subject of study of clinical, occupational and environmental toxicology. Toxic trauma, however, is the result of acute exposure to hazardous substances that cause life-threatening, seriously disabling acute effects and the intermediate effects that follow. Such life-threatening injury requires early recognition and life-support measures, as well as antidote and other supportive therapy.

3.4 The Classification of Toxic Hazards

Knowledge of the range and properties of toxic hazards is essential for the management of toxic trauma firstly to understand the presenting and possibly developing conditions in the patient and secondly to assess and understand the potential risks to emergency medical teams from transmission of the hazard.

Conventionally, toxic hazards are divided between those found in warfare and in industry. However, it should be noted that some agents have uses in both settings.

3.4.1 Toxic Industrial Chemicals

There are over 60 million catalogued chemical compounds, which is a reflection of the massive expansion of chemistry and chemical engineering over the past 150 years. Many of these compounds are immediately toxic and all are toxic in some respect depending on dose. Of these, there are now over 160,000 commercially available chemicals which reflect the expansion of the chemical industry over the same time period. About 70,000 industrial chemicals are routinely transported each year in the UK. Some 5000 chemicals have reliable medical toxicology information for acute and chronic exposure, most of it derived from animal studies.

Toxic agents which come from an industrial origin are known as TIC. These may be used as intermediaries in chemical syntheses or be designed to be toxic in their own right, as in the case of pesticides. TIC are carefully controlled during production and transport by a UN-based hazardous materials system (HAZMAT) which both classifies and identifies a toxic substance. TIC are classified into nine different classes and are identified by a code number. These are most familiar from the plates on the backs of lorries transporting toxic chemicals (Fig. 3.1). The classes of the HAZMAT system are shown in Box 3.1. HAZMAT provides a valuable way for emergency services to identify toxic agents to which casualties have been exposed, thus identifying essential physical and toxicological data which allow early and effective management of the incident and the patient.

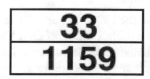

Fig. 3.1 A simple Kemmler plate. The *upper number* (repeated twice to emphasise its nature) is the class number of the compound (flammable liquid). The *lower number* is the international identification code for the compound—isopropyl ether. The exact form of the plate varies according to national practice

Box 3.1 The HAZMAT classification of toxic industrial chemicals
Class hazard classification:

1. Explosives
2. Pressurised gases
3. Flammable liquids
4. Flammable solids
5. Oxidising agents
6. Toxic substances
7. Radioactive substances
8. Corrosive substances
9. Miscellaneous dangerous substances

Toxic trauma from TIC is usually a result of accidental release, but in recent years, there have been growing concerns that chemicals being transported could be released deliberately as a result of terrorist action. Appendix A lists the properties of a range of TIC which are in common industrial use together with their HAZMAT identification numbers.

TIC are often stockpiled as feedstocks for the manufacturing of other compounds. Most damage from them is due to accidental release which may be in a gaseous or vapour or liquid form.

Within the HAZMAT classification, there are five main groups of TIC which cause toxic trauma:

1. Lung-damaging agents such as phosgene and chlorine (both of which have been used as CW agents and are used as intermediaries for other syntheses). Other compounds in this class include ammonia and fluorine
2. Chemical asphyxiants such as hydrogen cyanide and arsine
3. Sulphur compounds: H_2S and SO_2
4. Corrosive compounds: acids and bases
5. OP and carbamate pesticides

3.4.2   Military Toxic Hazards: Agents of Chemical Warfare

Military toxic hazards are termed CW agents. These are sometimes chemically identical or similar to some TIC but differ in their classification in that they are designed to be used by deliberate release to cause harm as opposed to the harm caused by industrial chemicals from accidental release.

Military agents are conventionally classified according to six classes of agents which are shown in Box 3.2.

> **Box 3.2 Classification of CW agents**
>
> 1. Nerve agents
>   Examples: sarin (GB), tabun (GA), soman (GD), VX, cyclosarin
> 2. Incapacitating agents
>   Examples: BZ, agent 15, LSD, opiate 'knockdown agents'
> 3. Chemical asphyxiants (agents blocking cellular respiration)
>   Hydrogen cyanide, cyanogen chloride and bromide
> 4. Lung-damaging agents
>   Chlorine, phosgene
> 5. Irritating (riot-control) agents
>   Examples: CS gas, CR gas
> 6. Vesicant (blistering) agents
>   Examples: mustard gas, lewisite

The physical properties of a number of CW agents are listed in Appendix B.

Although many compounds have been investigated for use as CW agents compared with TIC, the current spectrum of military hazards contains fewer compounds which are specifically designed to cause harm in battle. Many come from classes of compounds which are also found in TIC (e.g. lung-damaging agents such as phosgene and chlorine). Broadly, however, CW agents are more toxic than TIC. Because of the limited numbers of agents identified and in some cases produced and stockpiled, specific medical responses have been developed by the military to these toxic hazards which can be used on the battlefield.

Traditionally, there has been a separation of the classification of military and civil toxic hazards. However, the use of military hazards in the civil setting by terrorists and the confirmed use of chemical weapons against civilians during the Syrian Civil War make the integration of the two groupings of toxic compounds valuable in terms of emergency medical management.

3.5 Classification of Toxic Hazards According to Their Effects on Body Systems

It may not always be obvious what chemical agent has caused injury in a presenting patient. In terms of clinical recognition and management, an alternative way of classifying acute toxic hazards is to consider the effects they have on one or more somatic systems that may be affected after exposure. There will be reliance on toxidromes (see Chap. 5) which are agent class-specific rather than agent-specific in terms of the damage they cause to body systems.

3.5.1 Central Nervous System

Some toxic agents act on the central nervous system (CNS) producing effects at both the higher cortical and brainstem levels ranging from defective higher cognition, as in the case of incapacitating agents, or lower respiratory control, as in the case of organophosphate and opiate knockdown agents.

CW agent classes with a direct action on the CNS include nerve agents and incapacitating agents. TIC with central effects include organophosphate and carbamate pesticides and aliphatic hydrocarbons (including volatile general anaesthetics).

3.5.2 Peripheral Nervous System

Toxic agents which affect the peripheral nervous system do so through effects on the synapses of both the autonomic and voluntary systems and by direct actions on peripheral nerves. Military examples include nerve agents and toxins. Civil examples include pesticides and many marine and animal toxins.

3.5.3 Respiratory System

A wide range of toxic agents, both CW and TIC, have primary effects on the respiratory system, including airways and breathing. CW agents acting on the respiratory system include the lung-damaging agents, a wide range of toxic agents, both CW and TIC, chlorine, phosgene, organophosphate compounds and also inhaled vesicant agents such as mustard gas at high ambient temperatures.

TIC include lung-damaging agents (chlorine and phosgene are both used widely in the chemical industry), perfluoroisobutylene (PFIB) and isocyanates. All these compounds can lead to toxic pulmonary oedema at the alveolar level. In addition, there are many respiratory irritant agents which cause effects on the upper airways such as ammonia and hydrogen chloride and agents such as sulphur dioxide and toluene diisocyanate which cause severe bronchoconstriction.

3.5.3.1 Asphyxiants

These agents act on the respiratory system, both in the lungs and at the cellular respiratory level to cause hypoxia. Asphyxiants can be classified as:

1. Simple: an agent that displaces oxygen from the lungs causing a lowered absorption into the blood. Examples include carbon dioxide and nitrogen.
2. Chemical: an agent which prevents the transport to or use of oxygen in the cells thus interfering with aerobic respiration. Examples include carbon monoxide,

which combines with haemoglobin preventing it transporting oxygen to the cells, and hydrogen cyanide, which blocks the use of oxygen at the mitochondria in the cells thus blocking aerobic cellular respiration.

3.5.4 Heart and Central Vascular System

A number of toxic agents have a primary effect on the heart and blood vessels either directly or through disruption of nervous control. Examples include OP (both nerve agents and pesticides) and plant alkaloids such as atropine. These agents can cause life-threatening cardiac dysrhythmia with, again, terminal failure of cellular oxygen delivery. Military examples include nerve agents and toxins. Civil examples include pesticides and aliphatic hydrocarbons. In addition to TIC, there are a wide range of animal toxins, particularly from snakes which produce coagulopathies.

3.5.5 Alimentary System

Actions of toxic agents on the alimentary system are widely seen in cases of ingested self-poisoning. Although not a common route of exposure in the military setting, there are many reported cases in the civil setting. Civil examples include toxins (including ingested agricultural toxins such as ergotamine and mycotoxins) and pesticides. The outbreak of organophosphate poisoning as a result of using contaminated cooking oil which occurred in Morocco in the 1950s remains a classic example of ingested mass poisoning.

3.5.6 Skin and Epithelial System

Toxic agents affecting the skin and epithelial systems, in particular the eyes, may either act directly through corrosive actions, as in the case of acids or alkalis, or cause damage through actions on DNA and protein synthesis.

CW examples include vesicant agents which include mustard agents and lewisite, and toxins including mycotoxins, ricin and abrin. Note that CW vesicant agents have no equivalent in industrial use. They were developed solely to cause harm in warfare.

TIC examples include corrosive agents such as sulphuric acid and ammonia and a wide range of compounds that can cause acute dermatitis.

3.5.6.1 Irritant Agents

Some agents acting on the skin, eyes and epithelial membranes are classified as irritant compounds. An irritant is defined as a compound that causes inflammation of the skin and mucous membranes (including the nose, eyes and respiratory tract) and lachrymation. A wide range of TIC can be classed as irritant compounds. In the civil order setting, irritant gases such as CS and CR are used as riot-control agents. These agents are not, however, classed as CW agents since they have a wide safety margin (the ratio of the effective to the lethal dose) and are not subject to international CW treaties.

3.6 Properties of Toxic Chemical Agents

While being classified separately, both CW and TIC have many common properties. Although conditions in a battlefield and a civil setting are very different, the principles of management of casualties from CW and TIC are essentially the same, and there is a common approach to management of toxic trauma caused which is determined by the physical and biological properties of the agents.

The properties and actions of toxic agents are determined by the state in which they are released and by their physical and pathological characteristics. For each toxic chemical agent, four key properties can be defined, which are physical form, persistency, toxicity and latency of action. Of these, physical form and persistency are governed by the physical properties of the agent, and toxicity and latency are the biological properties.

3.6.1 Physical Properties of Toxic Chemical Agents

A basic understanding of the forms and physical properties of toxic hazards and the way they are dispersed is essential to the safe management of toxic releases and the casualties they have produced. Toxic hazards can exist in five physical forms. These are as follows:

Solid
Liquid
Vapour
Gas
Other airborne forms (aerosol, smoke, dust, mist)

Solid agents are those whose physical form conforms to specific dimensions. Solids are usually dispersed in the form of particles which can cause toxic trauma either externally or internally. Solids may stick to the body and to clothing and do not disperse easily.

Liquids exist in dynamic equilibrium with vapour that the liquid produces. Toxic trauma may therefore be caused by direct contact with the liquid or by inhalation of the vapour it produces.

Vapours are the gaseous phase above a volatile liquid. Vapours are gases whose critical temperature (the temperature above which a gas cannot be liquefied by applying pressure) is above room temperature. Essential characteristics of vapours are shown in Box 3.3.

Box 3.3 Characteristics of vapours

Vapour pressure This is defined as the partial pressure of the vapour in the atmosphere above a volatile liquid. Vapour pressure is temperature-dependent. The higher the temperature, the greater the vapour pressure. When vapour pressure reaches atmospheric pressure, boiling occurs. The importance of vapour pressure is that it gives an indication of the inhalational hazards from a toxic agent that is in a liquid state. Generally, a material with a low vapour pressure will not pose an inhalation hazard unless the patient is exposed to the material as an aerosol, in a confined space, for a prolonged period.

Vapour density This property characterises the vapour as being heavier or lighter than air. This indicates therefore whether there will be residual concentrations in low-lying areas around the site of the release.

A *gas* is a substance that is in a gaseous state at standard temperature and pressure (STP). The term vapour refers to the gaseous state of a chemical that is usually a liquid or solid at STP.

Apart from vapours and gases, toxic agents may also exist in mixed airborne states as follows:

An *aerosol* is a suspension of solid or liquid particles in a gas such as air. Smoke, fumes and dusts are airborne suspensions of solid particles, i.e. solid aerosols. Mists and fogs are airborne suspensions of liquid particles, i.e. liquid aerosols.

Smoke is a solid particulate aerosol formed by incomplete combustion of organic materials whose combustion also produces gases such as carbon monoxide and carbon dioxide.

Fumes are tiny solid particles formed by heating or vaporisation, and oxidation, of a metal. These microscopic metal oxide particles then condense in the air. Fume particles are usually less than or equal to 1–2 microns in diameter. This size of particle is readily respirable and reaches the air sacs (alveoli) of the lungs.

Dusts are solid particles suspended in air. These solid particles have been produced by some mechanical processes such as blasting, crushing, pulverising, drilling, grinding or abrading. Dusts can be toxic, fire or explosion hazards.

Mists are liquid droplets suspended in the air. Mists are generated by mechanically breaking up and dispersing a liquid by splashing, foaming or atomising.

Fog is formed by vapour condensation and is a visible suspension of fine droplets of liquid in a gas, e.g. clouds in the sky.

These physical states determine whether a toxic hazard (1) is a risk to the respiratory system, (2) can enter the body through the skin and (3) requires decontamination following exposure.

Because toxic trauma may be developing silently when the patient is first seen in or before hospital, it is important for physicians to have a basic knowledge of the physical states and properties of the toxic substances that may have been released. This will help predict the development and outcome of toxic injury.

3.6.2   Persistency

This is a measure of how long a released liquid or sold toxic agent will remain on the ground and present a continuing hazard. Chemical agents are divided into persistent and non-persistent agents. Persistent agents may be in a liquid or solid form. By contrast, non-persistent agents are vapours or gases which disperse quickly. Non-persistent agents have a low boiling point and a high vapour pressure (if a vapour). They act entirely through the respiratory tract. In contrast, persistent agents have a high boiling point and a low vapour pressure. Such agents have a persistency dependent upon climatic conditions and require responders to be wearing protective equipment. Examples of short-persistency toxic agents (which do not require decontamination) are hydrogen cyanide and other gases. Liquid agents such as nerve agents have a relatively high volatility with a high vapour pressure. Sarin has a volatility similar to water. The requirement for decontamination depends on the climatic conditions and the level of contamination. Long-persistency agents include the nerve agent VX, mustard gas and a wide range of liquid TIC. Box 3.4 presents some examples.

Box 3.4 Persistency of toxic chemical hazards

Chemical warfare agents

Short:
   Hydrogen cyanide
   Chlorine
   Sarin

Long:

    Cyanogen chloride and bromide
    Phosgene (relatively, due to its vapour density)
    Mustard gas
    Lewisite

Toxic industrial chemicals

Short:
    Sulphur dioxide
    Nitrogen oxides
    Ammonia

Long:
    Liquid chlorine
    Sulphuric acid
    Toluene diisocyanate

Non-persistent agents have a low boiling point and a high vapour pressure (if a liquid). They act entirely through the respiratory tract. In contrast, persistent agents have a high boiling point and a low vapour pressure.

In practical terms, knowledge of whether a substance is persistent or non-persistent is essential in assessing the risks to medical responders at the scene of the toxic release and also the dangers of transmission of a toxic substance from patients who have been brought undecontaminated to the hospital.

Importantly, persistency determines the requirement for decontamination after chemical exposure.

The essential danger associated with toxic agents having long persistency is that the toxic hazard will remain on the victim and in the surrounding area following exposure and may be transmitted to others further down the casualty evacuation line including those working in hospital emergency departments. This was the case following the release of the nerve agent sarin in the Tokyo metro in 1995 where a large number of medical and nursing staff themselves became casualties (see Chap. 10).

If a toxic agent has a long persistency, it will be necessary to decontaminate the patient as quickly as possible (1) to reduce further absorption of the agent and (2) to avoid spreading the contamination. Decontamination is a process that can affect the speed and efficiency of the provision of medical care for toxic trauma. Specific details of the techniques and rationale of decontamination are given in Chap. 5.

3.6.3   Toxicity

Toxicity is an expression of the harm caused to an organism by a toxic substance. Toxicology is the study of toxicity. There are many subsections of toxicology, both experimental and clinical. The application of this science in the clinical setting is termed clinical toxicology. Other subsections include occupational and environmental toxicology. A basic understanding of toxicity and its measurement is essential to the understanding of toxic trauma and to provide a rational basis for its management. This section is intended to provide an introduction to toxicological concepts and the measurement of toxic effects for non-specialist readers. Further detailed information is available from specialised texts.

3.6.3.1   The Development of Toxicology

The science of toxicology started in the Middle Ages. Paracelsus (Box 3.5) made a fundamental discovery in the study of poisons that it is not the substance itself which possesses toxicity but the dose of it that is given (*Sola dosis facit venenum*). This was a recognition that all things can be toxic if given in large enough doses. This concept still holds today and is the basis of the dose–response relationship which is fundamental to modern toxicology. The implication from Paracelsus's dictum is that no substance is essentially poisonous in its own right. It is the dose that determines harm. The effects of substances as different as ethyl alcohol and oxygen are considered good examples. The difference between the socially beneficial and the toxic effects of alcohol is well recognised, and in low doses, it is well tolerated over long periods. Similarly, oxygen which is essential for the production of energy in the body and therefore for life itself can be toxic in the form of oxygen free radicals in the lung when given in high concentrations over a prolonged period as is sometimes a necessity in the intensive care unit. The nineteenth-century Spanish physician Matteo Orfila (Box 3.6) is regarded as being the founder of modern toxicology as a science. He studied the specific harmful effects that toxic substances have on specific organs of the body (known as target organs) and the nature of damage caused by particular poisonous substances.

Box 3.5 Paracelsus

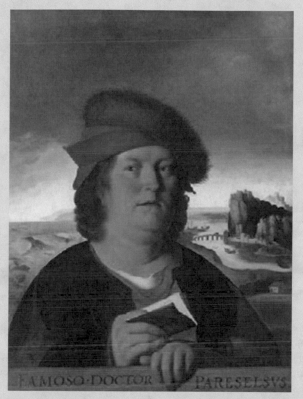

Source Wikimedia Commons, http://commons.wikimedia.org/wiki/File:Paracelsus.jpg

Paracelsus (born Philippus Aureolus Theophrastus Bombastus von Hohenheim, 1493–1541) was a German–Swiss alchemist who recognised the essential nature of toxic substances.

Of the nature of poisonous substances, Paracelsus wrote:

> *Alle Ding' sind Gift, und nichts ohn' Gift; allein die Dosis macht, daß ein Ding kein Gift ist.*
> *All things are poison, and nothing is without poison; only the dose permits something not to be poisonous.*

In other words, substances considered toxic are harmless in small doses, and conversely, an ordinarily harmless substance can be deadly if overconsumed.

Box 3.6 Matteo Orfila

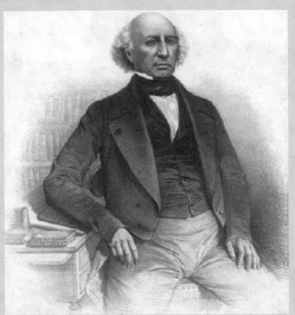

Source Wikimedia Commons, http://commons.wikimedia.org/wiki/File:Mathieu_Joseph_
Bonaventure_Orfila.jpg

Matteo Orfila (1787–1853) is regarded as the founder of modern toxicology. Although Spanish by origin, he worked largely in Paris, where, between 1814 and 1817, he published two major works *Traité des Poisons* and *Elements de Chimie Medicale* which earned him great recognition in the French scientific and medical communities. He was made Professor of the Faculty of Medicine in Paris in 1819 and subsequently held the highest positions in French medicine until the time of his death.

In the field of toxicology, he developed a systematic description of the effects of chemical substances on the human body. He studied the harm caused by poisons on specific organs and thus laid the basis for the modern target organ approach to poisoning.

3.6.3.2 Measuring Toxicity

The measurement of toxicity of substances in humans is difficult since planned prospective studies are essentially unethical. Information has therefore to be gathered from the study of accidental exposures or inferred from studies in animal models. This presents considerable difficulty due to differences in the way that various species respond to toxic substances. Humans respond in a variety of ways to toxic exposure. No single dose of a toxic substance will have exactly the same effect on different people. This is fundamental to the curve of effects on a population (the dose–response curve) which is a basic concept in toxicology (Fig. 3.2).

As noted previously, toxicity may be defined as the quantity of a toxic substance necessary to produce a harmful effect on any studied species. In the case of CW agents, this dose may be lethal or incapacitating in a short or medium term. For TIC, longer-term doses are defined (e.g. the dose that is immediately dangerous to life and health (IDLH) which is the concentration at which exposure must not exceed 30 min).

3.6.3.3 Expressing Toxicity

There are a number of terms used in both experimental and human toxicology which express the toxicity of a toxic substance. Here, we consider the standard expressions that may be encountered by clinicians. However, only a few of these are of value in direct clinical management where the amount of toxic agent that has caused the toxic effects cannot be measured with any accuracy. Most toxicological studies take place in animals, and the findings have to be interpreted in the human context. The principle value of most toxicological expressions in emergency medical responses to toxic trauma is to give an idea of the toxicity of the agent causing toxic trauma.

The following terms are used in describing exposure to a toxic agent:

Dose: The amount of any harmful substance that enters a living organism at a given time.

Exposure dose: The amount of the potentially harmful substance that is present in the environment or the source from which the harmful substance enters the living organism.

Absorbed dose: The exact amount of the potentially harmful substance that enters the living organism and is absorbed by it.

Administered dose: The amount of the potentially harmful substance that is administered to a living organism during experimental toxicology. Routes may be by mouth, injected or applied to the skin or given by inhalation as an aerosol or spray.

Target dose: The dose of a toxic substance that reaches a target organ.

Total dose: The sum of all individual doses, from all exposure routes.

Threshold dose: The dose at which a toxic effect is first observed or detected.

LD_{50}: The statistically derived dose at which 50 % of individuals will be expected to die (based on experimental observations, mostly in animals). This is the most frequently used estimate of the toxicity of substances.

LC_{50}: The calculated concentration of a gas lethal to 50 % of a group when exposure is inhalational.

There are a number of numerical ways of expressing toxicity in toxicology which are shown in Box 3.7.

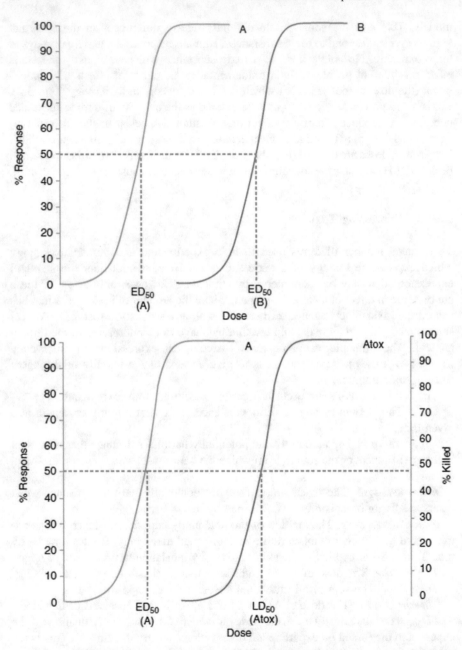

Fig. 3.2 Typical dose–response and toxicity curves. In the *upper* figure, both curves show variation in response to increasing doses of two substances A and B. Substance A is more potent than substance B because the ED_{50} (the dose that is effective in 50 % of the population) is lower. In the *lower* figure, the *right-hand curve* shows the toxic effects of A, and ED_{50} becomes LD_{50} (the dose causing death in 50 % of the population). The LD_{50} to ED_{50} ratio is known as the therapeutic index and indicates the margin of safety. (Credit from Baker et al. 2012, Fig. 1.3; by permission of Oxford University Press)

Box 3.7 Numerical expressions of toxicity

There are a number of terms used in both experimental and human toxicology which express the toxicity of a toxic substance. The standard expressions that may be encountered by clinicians are presented. However, only a few of these are of value in direct clinical management where the amount, e.g. inhaled, cannot be measured with any accuracy. The principle value in emergency responses to toxic trauma of most toxicological expressions is to give an idea of the toxicity.

The toxic dose (TD) is the dose that causes adverse or harmful effects. TD is expressed in a number of ways:

- TD_0 is the maximum dose that would cause harmful effects to 0 % of the population.
- TD_{10} is the dose that would cause harmful effects to 10 % of the population.
- TD_{50} is the dose that would cause harmful effects to 50 % of the population.
- TD_{90} is the dose that would cause harmful effects to 90 % of the population.

Although some accidental human toxicity data are available from CW and TIC agents, many values of toxicity in humans have been extrapolated from studies in animals.

It should be noted that increasing the concentration of inhaled agents causes a lowering of latency in many cases, as was seen in the first gas attack in World War I where there was clinical evidence of pulmonary oedema within a shorter time span than the usual 18–24 h.

3.6.3.4 Concentration × Time: The Haber Coefficient

For practical expressions of toxicity of inhaled toxic substances (the most common route for exposure to CW agents and TIC), the concentration × time product (Ct) is the most commonly presented expression of toxicity. The product is of concentration of the toxic agent in mg/m^3 and time in minutes. Ct is a commonly used and important expression of toxic trauma where the toxic agent is being inhaled. It is particularly valuable since most non-ingested toxicology is concerned with the inhalation of gases or vapours at a given concentration. Ct is usually expressed as $mg.min/m^3$ and is commonly known as the Haber coefficient after the German chemist Fritz Haber (Box 2.3) who first described it in relation to the inhaled CW agents used in the First World War. Initially, it was thought that a wide range of concentrations of gases inhaled for different times would be toxicologically equivalent, but we now know that this is not the case. Very low concentrations of hydrogen cyanide, for example, when inhaled over a long period do not have the same effects as high concentrations inhaled over a short space of time. This is because normal mechanisms of detoxification in the body remove low concentrations of the agent before they can reach toxic levels. In recent times, the concept of the Haber coefficient has been developed with the evolution of other more complex mathematical relationships. Box 3.8 shows a range of LCt_{50} values for commonly inhaled toxic agents.

Box 3.8 LCt_{50} values for some inhaled toxic chemical agents

Agent	LCt_{50} (mg min/m^3)
Chlorine	19,000
Phosgene	3,200
Methyl isocyanate	3,000
Hydrogen cyanide	1,500[a]
Tabun	400
Sarin	70

[a]Note that the value for HCN depends considerably on the exposure time, since HCN due to metabolism in the body over long exposures. This provides one important illustration of variation from the Haber principle

---

Despite its limitations, the coefficient is a useful assessment tool for acute toxic inhalations, particularly of CW agents like sarin which may have been used in a terrorist attack. An emergency physician, for example, armed with a knowledge of the approximate concentration levels at a point of release and the amount of time the victim had been exposed can predict potential toxic actions even if a toxidrome is not yet apparent. The most commonly used Ct expression is Ct_{50}. This is the Ct value at which signs and symptoms occur in 50 % of an exposed population. Use is also made of the LCt_{50} which is the Ct value that is fatal in 50 % of an exposed population. It is very important to note, however, that there is a fundamental difference between an LD_{50} and an LCt_{50} value. The former is a dose (usually measured in experimental animal models), whereas the latter describes an exposure. Exposure does not equal dose. The amount entering the body through the lungs at any ambient concentration will be a function of how fast the exposed person is breathing (the minute volume).

The Haber coefficient can be standardised for a set minute volume (10 l/min) with normal activity. The minute volume must be stated when quoting Ct values. If the minute volume is not specified, Ct is only an exposure and not an absorbed dose.

Since the original expression of the Ct index by Haber, there have been several complex modifications which are presented in Box 3.9 for readers who may require more detailed information. At the present time, the original equation $Ct = W$ has now been replaced by the expression $C^n t = W$, where n is a constant which varies between 1 and 7. In general, the more irritant the compound inhaled, the higher the value of n.

Box 3.9 Developments of the Haber principle

The limitations of the original simple expression of the Haber principle have been the subject of extensive study in recent years and revised expressions have been developed which overcome the failure of the original concept over long periods of exposure to low concentrations. The work can be summarised as follows:

(1) The original Ct index worked well for compounds producing irreversible effects by local reaction (e.g. chlorine and phosgene) or for compounds where the half-life for detoxification or elimination is long compared with the exposure time

(2) For some compounds such as hydrogen cyanide, the rate of detoxification and elimination prevent accumulation in the tissues until a certain inhaled threshold concentration is reached when the rate of uptake exceeds the rate of removal. Accumulation of the inhaled toxic substance then proceeds at a rate which is dependent on the difference between the inhaled concentration and the threshold concentration (i.e. the rate of uptake and a constant rate of removal). A modified Haber equation was produced by Flury and Zernik as early as 1931 which contained an 'elimination factor (e)' to modify the original equation to $(C - e)t = W$

(3) However, the Flury and Zernik equation does not itself hold for gases such as carbon monoxide which are taken up <u>and</u> excreted at the same time by the respiratory system nor for others such as HCN

(4) Carbon monoxide uptake is determined by the difference between the inhaled concentration and that in the body. This can be expressed by the exponential relationship $C(1 - e^{-tk}) = W$. This equation has been elaborated further into a set of complex equations which are beyond the scope of this book. However, for <u>high</u> concentrations of CO over a short space of time the uptake is approximately linear. This is the case when the blood concentration is 40 %, i.e. lethal over a short space of time which is the observed situation in many CO inhalation emergencies

(5) The pathological effects of the inhaled substance have an effect themselves on the Haber coefficient. In the case of HCl, the acid gas causes a reflex decrease in the respiratory rate (especially in mice). Conversely, HCN causes an initial reflex stimulation in respiration resulting in an increase in minute volume and an increase in HCN uptake and plasma concentration

(6)   The concentration of the inhaled substance is also found to affect the
      Haber coefficient. For HCN, the time to incapacitation is highly depen-
      dent on concentration. As a comparison, the Ct product for incapacitation
      (loss of consciousness) is 270 ppm min (parts per million.minute) at an
      inhaled concentration of 300 ppm, whereas at an inhaled concentration of
      87 ppm the Ct product is 2610 ppm min. In general the original Haber
      principle holds for the inflammatory effects of irritant gases such as HCl
      and for the non-lethal effects of lower concentrations of HCN
(7)   As a general rule concerning deviations from the Haber principle, high
      inhaled concentrations are considered more dangerous up to a given Ct
      level than lower concentrations
(8)   The safe levels of exposure to inhaled substances over a set period of time
      have been determined from animal and clinical toxicology data and are
      known as Acute Exposure Guideline Levels. These can be consulted via
      the Internet at https://www.epa.gov.aegl

3.6.3.5   Factors Affecting Toxicity

Absorption Rapid absorption of a toxic substance will have a more toxic effect than
a slowly absorbed poison that never reaches a toxic concentration. Many factors
influence the absorption of toxic agents.

Duration of Exposure The duration of exposure is another important determinant
of toxicity. The shorter the exposure time, the lower the absorbed dose and the less
the toxicity.

Exposure time frames can be described as acute or chronic. An acute exposure
usually refers to a high-dose, single exposure occurring over less than 24 h.

Chronic exposures are low-dose exposures occurring over a longer period,
usually a month or more. These exposures usually occur in the workplace.
Symptom onset with chronic (long-term) exposures can be confusing because there
is no clear event producing characteristic signs and symptoms.

Distribution Once a hazardous material is absorbed, it passes into the blood
stream and distributes throughout the body. For example, carbon monoxide is
distributed in the bloodstream, bound to haemoglobin as carboxyhaemoglobin.
Many factors influence the distribution of a hazardous material, including water
solubility versus lipid solubility. An example is found in organophosphate insecticides which are concentrated in fat tissue and continuously released with time,
allowing them to redistribute to the nervous system.

Metabolism (Catabolism) Metabolism of absorbed toxic agents usually takes
place in the liver, but can also occur in the kidneys and lungs. There are two main

types of metabolism, anabolism and catabolism. Toxicology is essentially concerned with the latter.

For many toxic agents, no specific measures exist to prevent metabolism once the materials are absorbed. This highlights the importance of preventing or mitigating exposure through protection.

Elimination Some toxic agents are not metabolised and are eliminated from the body unchanged. Examples include the simple asphyxiant nitrogen or the systemic asphyxiant carbon monoxide. A major route of elimination for almost all gases and most vapours is via the lungs. In other words, they are eliminated through their route of entry. This highlights the importance of ensuring adequate pulmonary ventilation and oxygenation for patients exposed to inhaled toxicants.

The other main excretory organs are the liver and the kidneys. Hepatic metabolism may result in polar metabolites that are more water-soluble than the parent chemical, so they are more easily eliminated in the urine. The liver also excretes non-polar and less water-soluble metabolites into the bile, with subsequent elimination in the faeces.

The kidneys eliminate polar, water-soluble compounds and polar, water-soluble metabolites into the urine. Haemodialysis is used in clinical toxicology if the patient has kidney (renal) failure or to enhance elimination of toxic metabolites of poisons.

3.6.4   Latency

Toxic agents produce their effects in the body with a variable time following exposure. The period of delay between the appearance of effects and the exposure is termed latency. Although latency is a very important factor in the presentation and management of toxic trauma, it has not been investigated nearly as much as toxicity. Normally, latencies are expressed crudely in minutes or hours for acute exposures. Longer-term latencies of days or even months are possible with some sequelae to toxic exposure. Long-term neuropathy following OP exposure and carcinogenesis following mustard gas exposure are examples. Given that latency will, like toxicity, be subject to biological variation in any population, a reasonable way of expressing it would be as an L_{50} value, but inexplicably this has not been the case so far. Toxic hazards may be subclassified according to the latency of the appearance of the effects they produce as being short or long latency.

3.6.4.1   Short Latency

Short-latency acute toxic hazards are defined as chemical substances which cause toxic trauma over a short period after exposure. Effects will be revealed within seconds to minutes. Short-latency toxic hazards produce effects that require the use of emergency life-support procedures and/or specific antidotes. Examples include nerve agents and hydrogen cyanide. Some compounds have a dual latency (such as phosgene) with the onset time of pulmonary oedema dependent on the initial exposure of the dose received.

3.6.4.2   Long Latency

Compounds in this class cause toxic trauma within hours to days following a single exposure. In some cases, there may be dual latency with early signs and symptoms followed by the development of other life-threatening conditions some hours later.

Examples of compounds that fall into this class are mustard gas and lung-damaging compounds such as methyl isocyanate and chlorine. It is important to distinguish acute long-latency toxic effects from toxic effects that arise from chronic low-level exposure to a toxic chemical. Lead poisoning is an example. Compounds in this class may be regarded as producing long-term chronic poisoning rather than toxic trauma with long latency which follows acute exposure. Box 3.10 shows examples of short- and long-latency acute toxic hazards.

Box 3.10 Examples of short- and long-latency toxic chemical agents

Chemical warfare agents

Short latency:
  Nerve agents: e.g. sarin
  Lung-damaging agents (initial irritating actions): e.g. chlorine, phosgene, hydrogen cyanide

Long latency:
  Lung-damaging agents (secondary actions producing toxic pulmonary oedema)
  Vesicant agents: e.g. mustard gas

Toxic industrial agents

Short latency:
  Irritant gases: e.g. sulphur dioxide, oxides of nitrogen
  Corrosive agents: e.g. sulphuric acid, sodium hydroxide
  Toluene diisocyanate

Long latency:
  Methyl isocyanate, producing toxic pulmonary oedema

In the clinical management of toxic trauma, awareness of latency is of great importance. Many CW agents and incapacitating agents (also knockdown agents) have short latency to maximise their effects in a battlefield. Nerve agents and chemical asphyxiants such as hydrogen cyanide fall into this category and rapidly produce characteristic signs and symptoms (toxidromes) which aid diagnosis and treatment. Toxic agents with longer latency present a problem clinically in that the damage caused by an exposure may not be apparent at the time when the patient is first clinically examined. The latency of production of pulmonary oedema by lung-damaging agents such as phosgene and the effects of sulphur mustard gas are examples.

3.7   Conclusions

In this chapter, we have outlined the ways of classifying the very large number of toxic chemicals that exist in both civil and military settings. An understanding of classification of compounds is important in the early recognition of a toxic hazard that may have produced toxic trauma. Equally, a basic understanding of the physical and biological properties that characterise them is important in the management of casualties.

Further Reading

Baker DJ, Karalliedde L, Murray VSG, Maynard Rl, Parkinson NHT (eds) (2012) Essentials of toxicology for health protection: hand book for health professionals, 2nd edn. Oxford University Press, Oxford, UK
Marrs TC, Maynard RL, Sidell FR (eds) (2007) Chemical warfare agents: toxicology and treatment. John Wiley and Sons Ltd, Chichester, UK
Tuorinsky SD, Sciuto A (2008) Toxic inhalational injury and toxic industrial chemicals. In: Tuorinsky SD (ed) Medical aspects of chemical warfare. Office of the Surgeon General, US Army. Borden Institute, Washington DC, USA pp 339–370 (Chap. 10)
Maynard Rl, Purser DA (2016) Haber's Law and its application to combustion products. Purser D, Maynard RL (eds) Royal Society of Chemistry, London UK

Chapter 4
Exposure to Toxic Hazards

Abstract Exposure to the toxic hazards considered in the previous chapter can occur in a variety of ways, both accidental and deliberate. The form of exposure and the circumstances, such as whether the release is in the open air or in a confined space, determines the degree of toxic trauma caused. This chapter considers the ways in which toxic exposure can occur, how toxic releases are detected and identified and how to reduce secondary exposure of emergency teams by the use of personal protection equipment and decontamination. Because of the dangers presented to emergency responders, a clear understanding of these points forms an essential basis to reacting to chemical incidents and the safe management of casualties. Training in the use of protective equipment and decontamination is essential for the safe conduct of pre-hospital and hospital management of toxic trauma.

4.1 Introduction

Toxic trauma from exposure to released toxic agents is a relatively rare event compared with individual accidental or deliberate poisoning. Risks exist to populations which are dependent upon local circumstances such as war or terrorist attack or from the proximity of industrial chemical plants. This chapter concerns with the ways in which exposure to toxic chemical agents can occur, and how it can be detected and mitigated by the use of personal protective equipment (PPE) and decontamination procedures. An understanding of the nature of toxic releases is of great importance to medical responders dealing with casualties with toxic trauma. Unlike physical trauma where the originating event such as an explosion is not usually a hazard for responders, the persistent nature of some toxic chemicals makes their release a continuing hazard, not only for those already exposed but to responding emergency teams both on-site and further down the evacuation line, even into the hospital itself.

Exposure to toxic agents can occur both accidentally and deliberately. Individual self-poisoning is the presentation most familiar to emergency medical personnel. But apart from ingested poisoning, toxic exposure can take place via a number of other routes. The most important and common, particularly for mass exposure, is the respiratory route which applies to both chemical warfare (CW) agents and toxic industrial chemicals. The use of gases such as chlorine and phosgene in WWI and the release of methyl isocyanate from a factory in Bhopal, India, in 1984 provide classic examples.

4.2   Acute and Chronic Exposures

Exposure time frames can be described as acute or chronic. Acute exposure to a toxic agent may be defined as an immediate release and exposure to a toxic substance over a period of minutes up to 24 h which gives rise to short latency somatic toxic effects. Chronic exposures may be defined as low-dose exposures occurring over a longer period, usually a month or more. These may occur in the workplace or from living near an industrial facility. Symptom onset with chronic (long term) exposures can be confusing because there is no clear temporal link between an exposure and the development of disease. Chronic exposures may give rise to diseases that have no clear toxidrome (see Chap. 5) or may be carcinogenic in nature. Acute exposures lead to specific collections of signs and symptoms developing within a relatively short space of time and which give rise to specific manifestations of toxic trauma. Chronic exposure to low levels of toxic substances can cause diseases which are the concern of public health practitioners and clinical toxicologists. Toxic trauma, as defined in Chap. 1, concerns the immediate and continuing consequences of an individual or collective exposure to an acute single release of a toxic agent.

4.3   Routes of Exposure to Toxic Agents

4.3.1   Inhalation

Inhalation is the most frequently encountered route of exposure for both CW agents and toxic industrial chemicals. Toxic substances can enter the body through inhalation of gases, vapours, smoke, fumes, dusts, mists or fog. The properties of these were described in the previous chapter. Following inhalation, toxic substances can cause trauma at all levels of the respiratory tree and in the lung parenchyma before being absorbed into the circulation where further damage can occur.

Following the first gas attacks in 1915, filtration respirators were quickly developed to filter out the toxic substance before it was inhaled (Fig. 4.1). This approach is still used by armies around the world up to the present day. In a trained and organised military setting where toxic hazards are recognised through intelligence and can be detected using a variety of means continuing to operate in a contaminated area, using special protective equipment is possible. In the civil setting where exposure to an inhaled toxic agent is usually unexpected, the best way

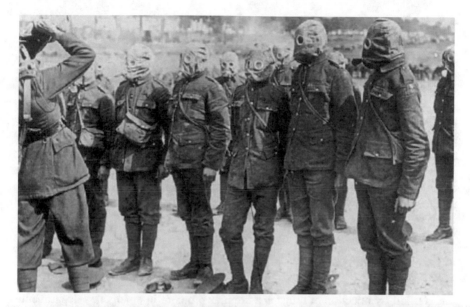

Fig. 4.1 World War I gas masks. (Photograph reproduced by courtesy of the National Archives)

to alter absorption via inhalation is to remove the patient as quickly as possible from the source of exposure. Simple measures such as ensuring adequate ventilation of an enclosed space will reduce the concentration of the released gas or vapour and thus the exposure dose to the patient. Inhaled exposure risk is greatly increased in confined spaces such as underground railway stations and tunnels due to the higher concentrations of agent that can be achieved.

4.3.2 Skin and Mucous Membranes

Many toxic agents are absorbed through the skin and mucous membranes, including the eyes. The skin has a large surface area. Intact skin provides a barrier to many, but not all toxic agents. With skin contact, some substances such as mustard gas and corrosive chemicals such as sulphuric acid and sodium hydroxide cause dermal damage at the point of contact. Other compounds such as nerve gases easily pass through the skin and cause initially local and then systemic effects. Skin absorption of toxic agents is increased in cases of skin damage or in hot environments. Certain areas of the body are more susceptible to percutaneous chemical absorption than others. For instance, the genital area will absorb chemicals such as mustard gas many times faster than the hand or foot.

4.3.3   Ingestion

Toxic agents can also enter the body by ingestion. Intentional ingestions usually occur in suicidal adults but accidental adult ingestions can occur due to poor hand washing prior to eating or smoking, or by swallowing concentrated toxic solutions Accidental ingestions occur most often in children. Mass ingestion of toxic agents has occurred where there has been industrial environmental contamination of the food supply. Examples include organophosphate poisoning due to contaminated cooking oil in North Africa in the 1950s and mercury poisoning in Minamata disease in Japan. However, most reported incidents of mass ingestion poisoning are chronic rather than acute in nature. An exception is the ingestion of bacterial toxins causing acute food poisoning.

4.3.4   Injection

Intoxication by injection of drugs is a familiar problem in emergency departments. However, it is less common in deliberate and accidental toxic agent release. There is a possibility of injection entry of hazardous materials following distribution by explosive device which causes shrapnel injury. In addition, contamination of open wounds by CW agents is a possibility that has been considered by the military for a number of years.

4.3.5   Envenomation

Envenomation is the most common form of natural exposure to toxic agents in the form of toxins. Toxin injection following bites by spiders and snakes and sea creatures occurs worldwide, and procedures for management involving life support and antitoxins are well developed. However, a number of toxins which appear in nature and which are usually active by subcutaneous or intramuscular injection have been considered for use as CW agents. There are reports that a number of these, including botulinum toxin, may be active when absorbed through the respiratory route (see Chap. 11). Box 4.1 shows a summary of the potential routes of exposure to toxic agents.

Box 4.1 Classification of the routes of exposure to toxic agents
Classification of exposures to toxic agents

1. Accidental, individual

   Ingestion
   Mistaken labelling of alimentary products
   Accidental overdose of prescription medicines
   Accidental ingestion of poisonous plants and animals
   Ingestion of food products contaminated with toxins
   Industrial contamination, e.g. cooking oils, Minamata disease
   Excessive ingestion of recreational agents (e.g. alcohol)

   Intramuscular/intravenous
   Accidental overdose of prescription drugs (e.g. insulin)
   Anaesthesia
   Ward/ICU
   Paediatric/adult

   Inhalational
   Deliberate release of CW agents
   Industrial releases
   Smoke inhalation
   Carbon monoxide inhalation
   Crop spraying
   Anaesthesia
   Nebulised drug delivery systems

2. Deliberate: individual/homicidal/self-poisoning

   Oral
   Self-poisoning

   Drugs
   Household products
   Industrial products
   Agricultural products
   Plants

   Homicidal poisoning
   IM/IV

   Tribal/ritual
   Snake pits
   Blow pipes and curare

Dermal and epithelial
Toxins

   aconitine
   mycothecenes
   ricin

3. Deliberate mass exposure

   Oral
   Ritual, tribal
   Terrorism—contamination of food and water supplies

   Inhalational
      Deliberate release of CW agents and toxic industrial chemical (TIC)
      CW and toxic terrorism
      A major route for the dissemination of agents of CW—airborne dissemination, spraying, shell burst, rocket launchers)
      Genocidal

HCN in mass exterminations during World War II

   Dermal

   Nerve agents
   VX
   Thickened soman (GD)

   Vesicant agents

   Mustard agents
   Lewisite

   Toxins

   T2 mycothecenes

   Oral

   Many CW agents act through the ingestion route particularly as a result of secondary contamination

4.4   Detection of Accidental and Deliberate Exposure to Toxic Chemical Agents

Detection of a released toxic agent is important both to confirm that a toxic hazard exists and to identify its nature so that the appropriate protection and treatment measures can be put in place. Detection may involve the body senses such as smell and sight and also the use of automated devices which can detect the released agent as a result of its physical and chemical properties. Detection of a chemical release is often confused with monitoring. Strictly, detection, as its name suggests, is the process by which a chemical agent release is revealed. Monitoring is the process of measuring the amount of released chemical that is present after the release, both in the atmosphere for non-persistent agents and on buildings and persons where the released agent is persistent.

4.4.1   Military

Detection and identification is an integral part of CW, and a wide range of technologies are used in the battlefield including mass spectroscopy and ion drift devices. Military detection devices are designed to give an alarm so that appropriate CW protection protocols can be followed. The UK Chemical Agent Monitor is an example of the latter which can detect contamination from nerve, cyanide and vesicant agents using ion drift technology. Although strictly a monitoring device, it has been used as a detector at sea during the First Gulf War (Fig. 4.2).

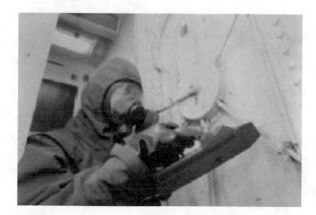

Fig. 4.2 The Chemical Agent Monitor (Smiths Detection Ltd, Watford, UK). This device can detect contamination by a range of CW agents, including nerve agents and sulphur mustard

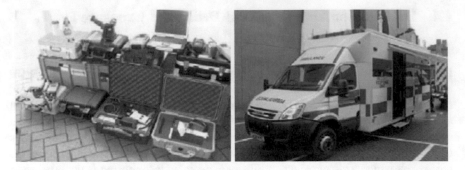

Fig. 4.3 The range of equipment carried by the British hazardous area paramedical response teams (HART)

4.4.2 Civil

In the civil setting, unlike the military, there are few preset detection and alarm systems in vulnerable public places such as the metro system. Toxic releases are usually the responsibility of the fire and rescue services who have their own detection equipment. Increasingly, primary emergency medical response teams also have their own equipment for detection and identification of a toxic agent release. Figure 4.3 shows the range of equipment carried by the British hazardous area paramedical response teams (HART).

In non-military toxic releases, detection relies on the use of the senses and recognition of unusual circumstances to indicate a toxic release. Box 4.2 summarises basic indications of a toxic agent release.

4.4.3 Identification of a Toxic Release by Medical Responders

The primary emergency responders to chemical incidents carry out a primary reconnaissance using equipment mentioned above. This may produce an immediate identification of the agent concerned. Eye witness accounts are also important and a possible pattern (toxidrome) of signs and symptoms in victims (see Chap. 6).

In addition, reports of the nature of the incident (e.g. was there an explosive or passive discharge) will be important as will be the nature of the location (open or closed release).

Box 4.2 Simple indicators of a toxic agent release: *Steps 1, 2, 3* **and bystander observation**

1. Standard triggers of a toxic release for emergency personnel (STEP) ambulance services use the following simple guidance to determine whether a toxic release may have taken place in the case of one or more casualties.

Step 1	One casualty	Approach using normal procedures
Step 2	Two casualties with identical signs and symptoms	Approach with caution, report arrival and send a situation report
Step 3	Three or more casualties with identical signs and symptoms	Do not go to the scene but to a perimeter rendezvous point and wait further instructions

2. Bystander observations indicating a toxic agent release

A chemical agent release should be considered if bystanders:

1. *See* a gas or vapour cloud
2. *Smell* anything unusual
3. *Hear* an explosive discharge followed by the deposition of droplets or splashes of liquid
4. *See* visible signs of toxic injury without any obvious physical cause of injury toxidromes in exposed persons or dead animals, fish or insects in the location

In addition, for accidental civil toxic releases, detailed information about the toxic agent may be quickly available from Kemmler plates on production sites and transporting vehicles (Sect. 3.4.1).

4.5 Mitigation of Exposure to Toxic Agents

Toxic trauma is made worse by the length of time to which the victim is exposed to the toxic agent. This is clear from the consideration of the Haber coefficient (Chap. 3) where the concentration of the released agent and the time of exposure are the factors. It is therefore essential that persons exposed to toxic agents are removed from the scene of the release as quickly as possible. In addition, it is essential to protect emergency responders from the action of the toxic agent which may still be present at the site of release or on the clothing of victims and which could be carried down the medical evacuation chain to the hospital emergency department and beyond, as was the case following the release of the nerve gas sarin in Tokyo in 1995 (Chap. 10).

The key stages in the reduction of toxic trauma both to the original victims and to responders are as follows:

1. Protection of emergency personnel to prevent them becoming the next casualties
2. Removal of the victims from the immediate release area
3. Decontamination of the released toxic agent, if it is persistent

4.6 Personal Protective Equipment

The identification and the risks presented by a released toxic agent may not be clear in the initial stages of an incident. Fire and emergency medical personnel responding to such incidents must therefore take appropriate steps to wear suitable personal protective equipment (PPE) to avoid becoming casualties themselves. As will be seen in the next chapter, incidents involving toxic releases are controlled by cordoning the surrounding area into hot, warm and cold (non-contaminated) zones. The hot zone, nearest the site of the release of the chemical, is where rescue operations to remove casualties are performed, usually by the fire services. Casualties are then taken to the warm zone where decontamination is performed if necessary before casualties can be transported onwards to the cold zone and ongoing medical care. The essential difference between the hot and warm zones is determined by the ambient concentration of the released toxic agent, with the greatest concentration being at the point of release.

Hot zone working has always been regarded as the job of the fire services who are equipped to face any degree of toxicity and corrosiveness presented by the released chemical. Firemen are used to wearing self-contained breathing apparatus (SCBA) supplied with air from bottles or airlines since they are exposed to carbon monoxide and smoke products of combustion as a regular hazard from firefighting. Importantly, carbon monoxide, a major toxic hazard of combustion, is not absorbed by filtration respirators.

In contrast to the civilian situation, the military have traditionally taken a different approach to PPE since carbon monoxide is not usually a battlefield hazard and self-contained breathing apparatus is not easily deployed in the field. Thus, military PPE uses relatively lightweight suits with filtration respirators where ambient air is filtered through a cartridge containing activated charcoal mixed with silver salts to remove cyanide. This approach has now been adopted by paramedical and medical teams in many countries for the following reasons:

1. The degree of secondary contamination on patients who have been removed from the hot zone is considerably less than the contamination at the point of release. This means that heavy, self-contained suits with SCBA are not necessary.
2. The use of lightweight suits allows essential life support and other medical care to be given early to victims by protected medical responders.

Box 4.3 shows the general classification of personal protective equipment.

Box 4.3 The classification of personal protective equipment

The classification of PPE	
Level A	Positive pressure self-contained breathing apparatus or a pressure-demand supplied respirator (air hose)
	Fully encapsulating chemical resistant suit (one piece)
	Double-layer chemical resistant gloves
	Chemical resistant boots
	Airtight seal between the suit, gloves and boots
Level B	Positive pressure self-contained breathing apparatus
	Chemical resistant long sleeve suit (two piece)
	Double layer of chemical resistant gloves
	Chemical resistant boots
Level C	Full-face filtration respirator
	Chemical resistant suit
	Chemical resistant outer gloves
	Chemical resistant boots
Level D	Full face respirator or filtration mask
	Usually normal working clothes

Level A PPE (Fig. 4.4) provides maximum protection against vapours and liquids which are toxic and corrosive.

Level B PPE is used when full respiratory protection is required but the danger to the skin from liquid contact is less. It differs from level A in that it uses a non-encapsulating, splash protective chemical resistant suit ('splash suit') that provides level A protection against liquids but is not airtight.

Fig. 4.4 Tokyo Fire
Department HAZMAT teams
wearing level A suits during
the 1995 Tokyo sarin release

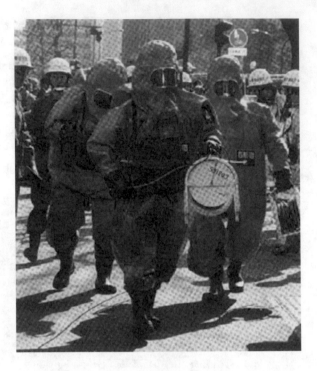

Level C PPE (Fig. 4.5) uses a lighter splash suit than level B and provides
respiratory protection by filtering the ambient atmosphere. It is used by several
emergency services to allow medical and paramedical responders to provide
emergency care inside a contaminated zone (Box 4.4).

Level C suits (Figs. 4.5, 4.6, 4.7) are regarded by many emergency medical
services in Europe as being suitable for operation by emergency medical services
personnel working in the warm zone to provide essential care to patients awaiting
and during decontamination (Fig. 4.6). The weight of the suits and thickness of the
gloves allows manoeuvrability and dexterity which permit essential medical operations such as inserting a pharyngeal airway or intubation and ventilation. While
levels A and B suits allow only about 20–30 min of breathing from a self-contained
air supply, filtration respirators can be used for considerably longer and the car-
tridges can be changed inside a contaminated zone using established procedures.

Fig. 4.5 GIAT level C
protection used by the Paris
Emergency Medical Service.
(Photograph courtesy of
SAMU de Paris)

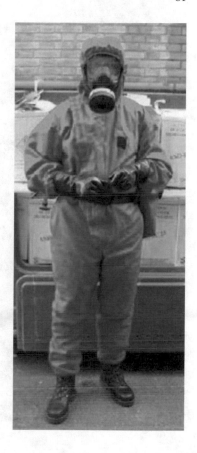

Heat stress, which is a serious disadvantage of level A and B PPE, is reduced in level C PPE and this can be improved further by the use of ventilated suits.

Box 4.4 Use of PPE by emergency medical personnel in France
In France, plans and equipment and training have been provided to allow the emergency medical service (SAMU) to work in the warm zone. The approach has been to use specially procured level C suits and a filtration respirator which allows good visual contact and speech transmission. SAMU emergency teams are medically led, and the doctor in charge is allowed clinical freedom in his choice of treatment options rather than following set protocols as in paramedical systems. This improves flexibility of clinical response in the difficult operating circumstances of the hot/warm zone. SAMU personnel received extensive training in wearing level C PPE and stocks of equipment are held and maintained in ambulance dispatching centres ready for immediate use by normal, on call emergency medical response teams. These

Fig. 4.6 Decontamination exercise by personnel wearing a Swedish level C suit. The filtration canisters for the respirator are belt mounted

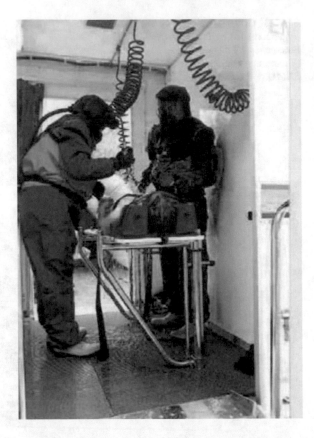

Fig. 4.7 British army soldier wearing a level C protective suit. The respirator is a military type S 10 with a CW filtration canister. Respirators have been used in military training and operations since the start of CW during the First World War

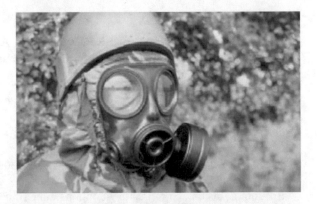

personnel are able to perform all the usual advanced life-support actions while wearing PPE, such as endotracheal intubation, artificial ventilation and peripheral intravenous vascular access.

4.7   Decontamination

Decontamination of the patient is necessary when a persistent toxic agent has been released and is present on the skin and clothing. The problems created by the need for decontamination in the context of the management of a hazardous materials (HAZMAT) incident are addressed in the next chapter. Here, we consider the basic techniques of individual and mass decontamination that should be understood by medical personnel.

4.7.1   Decontamination Basics

In the context of toxic chemical agents, decontamination may be defined as the removal of a persistent agent from a victim or his surrounding area in order to minimise further exposure and toxic trauma to both the victim and emergency responders. Box 4.5 shows the essential characteristics of basic decontamination.

Box 4.5 Characteristics of basic decontamination
Decontamination is the

- reduction or
- removal of any toxic agent.

  Decontamination can be:

- Applied to responders/personnel with or without PPE or to casualties/patients (ambulatory or not)
- Performed on-scene or at hospitals
- Performed by responders or as guided self-help
- Necessary for few or many persons (mass decontamination)
- External or internal
- Wet or dry
- Performed by different services (fire, medical)

  Decontamination may be accomplished by:

- Physical removal
- Dilution and elution by water
- (Chemical) neutralisation

  Decontamination

- reduces the spread of contamination,

  - e.g. to transport vehicles and

- protects the medical staff/facility.

4.7.1.1 Decontamination Techniques

These are divided between (1) dry and (2) wet.

Dry decontamination is favoured by the military who often do not have enough water available for wet decontamination. The technique uses clay, called Fullers Earth, to adsorb the toxic agent from the skin and clothing.

Wet decontamination is usually performed using copious quantities of water.

In case of individual decontamination, contamination is removed using a rinse–wipe–rinse sequence which can be aided by the use of liquid soft soap to reduce surface tension.

Mass decontamination is a technique favoured by fire services and other organisations that have responsibility for HAZMAT incident management. It is carried out in the warm zone (the zone of secondary contamination) to which contaminated casualties are moved following rescue (see Chap. 5).

Decontamination is performed either at the incident site in the warm zone as indicated or at the hospital emergency department inside a chemical decontamination facility which is set up outside the hospital building and which has a dedicated entry point to the further onward treatment in the emergency department.

4.7.2 Secondary Contamination

Chemical incidents pose a special risk to rescuers and hospitals since the spread of contamination to staff may adversely affect their performance and long-term health. There have been many reports on secondary contamination of healthcare staff and facilities during chemical incident response, sometimes as a result of a single contaminated patient. In the USA, it has been estimated that secondary contamination of healthcare staff occurs in 0.4 % of accidental industrial chemical incidents. In contrast, the deliberate release of chemicals is associated with a higher risk of spread of contamination due to a number of factors:

- The release may be covert.
- The possible larger numbers of casualties involved.
- The toxicity of the agents may be higher.

In the Tokyo subway attacks in 1995, 10–23 % of rescuers at the scene and hospital emergency staff displayed the clinical features of exposure to sarin. Some of these displayed chronic physiological abnormalities such as disturbed lymphocyte function 3 years later and cognitive impairment at least 7 years afterwards. In one instance, 11 doctors were significantly affected while treating two patients (one required treatment for seizures, the other received cardiopulmonary resuscitation for 40 min).

4.7.2.1 Factors Affecting Secondary Contamination

A number of factors determine the risk and severity of secondary contamination:

1. Physicochemical properties of the chemical, persistence and dispersion

The state of the chemical influences the risk of spread of contamination. Gases pose a low risk of secondary spread to healthcare staff because they disperse relatively rapidly once the patient has been removed from the source of exposure. Similarly, vapours usually present a low risk unless significant condensation has occurred on the skin. Liquids are more likely to spread because they are likely to persist on the patient until they reach medical attention. The risk is directly related to the volatility of the agent (rate at which is evaporates): A highly volatile substance presents an immediate danger when it is released but disperses quickly so it poses a relatively lower risk of spreading. A less volatile agent is more persistent and therefore is more likely to be present on the patients if they reach an emergency department. Environmental factors will influence the persistence and dispersion of chemical agents, thereby influencing the potential for exposures to occur. Hot, windy weather should encourage evaporation of volatile agents, thereby resulting in a relative reduction in the risk of emergency responders and hospital personnel being subjected to secondary contamination (although vasodilatation may occur under such conditions which may promote transcutaneous absorption for those exposed). Rainfall may also result in removal of some of the external contamination. In addition, the presence of water may enhance absorption through the skin with the resultant possibility of exacerbating toxic effects.

Both prevailing climatic and more transient weather conditions (such as wind direction and the presence or absence of a temperature inversion) may affect the dispersion of gaseous, vaporised or aerosolised agents. Local topography and the distribution of buildings will also influence air flow and agent dispersion.

2. Direct transmission by patients

This depends on the concentration and inherent toxicity of the chemical with which a patient is contaminated and the proximity and duration of contact with the staff. Chemical agents can be present on the patient's skin, hair and clothes, all of which can be reduced by external decontamination. However, certain volatile agents may also be present in exhaled breath ('respiratory off-gassing') and ingested chemicals may be present in vomitus, neither of which is removed by external decontamination. In these circumstances, regular rotation of staff away from the clinical areas may reduce the effects of secondary contamination.

Although water is likely to be the most readily used universal decontaminant, there are theoretical concerns on its efficacy. As previously noted, the transcutaneous absorption of agent such as sulphur mustard may be increased by water; similarly, the burns produced by concentrated acids may be exacerbated by the exothermic reaction produced when water is added. However, in practice, drenching casualties with water is likely to remove the contamination while minimising these adverse effects. The practical implication of this is that decontamination showers should have a relatively high flow rate. The effect of water temperature should also be noted; relatively lower temperatures may reduce vasodilatation of skin vessels (thereby inhibiting absorption), but the use of cold water increases the risk of hypothermia and is likely to discourage the patients from washing thoroughly.

4.8   Conclusions

Exposure to toxic agents may be acute or chronic. Toxic trauma is the result of an acute single exposure which gives rise to signs and symptoms within minutes or hours. Detection of an acute release can be done using simple observation of the circumstances or using special detection devices which are used by fire and rescue services and some emergency medical services.

Although there are many pathways for toxic agents to enter the body, the main danger for mass exposure is the respiratory route. Reduction of exposure in this way can be achieved by the use of personal protective equipment. The main component of this for medical emergency teams is a filtration respirator.

Mitigation of exposure can be achieved by removing the victim from the area of toxic release and by decontamination if the agent released is persistent. Many toxic gases do not fall into this category and do not require decontamination. Mass decontamination at toxic release sites is usually done by the fire and rescue services using showering but emergency medical services should be familiar with individual techniques of decontamination and be aware of the potential hazards faced from secondary contamination from contaminated patients.

Further Reading

Borak J, Callan M, Abbott W (1991) Hazardous materials exposure: emergency response and patient care. Prentice Hall, New Jersey

Bronstein AC, Currance PL (1994) Emergency care for hazardous materials exposure, 2nd ed. Mosby Lifeline

Clarke SFJ, Chilcott RP, Wilson JC et al (2008) Decontamination of multiple casualties who are chemically contaminated: a challenge for acute hospitals. Prehospital Disast Med 23(2): 175–181

Cocciardi JA (2004) Weapons of mass destruction and terrorism response: a field guide. Jones and Bartlett, London

Okumura T, Nomura T, Suzuki T et al (2007) The Dark Morning: the experiences and lessons learned from the Tokyo sarin attack In: Marrs Tc, Maynard RL, Sidell FR (eds) Chemical warfare agents: toxicology and treatment, chap 13. Wiley, Chichester

Rimpel LY, Boehm DE, O'Hern MR et al (2008) Chemical defense equipment. In: Tuorinsky SD (ed) Medical aspects of chemical warfare, chap 17. Office of the Surgeon General, US Army, Borden Institute, Washington, DC, pp 559–592

Chapter 5
Responding to Chemical Releases: Essentials of Organisation and Incident Management

Abstract Any release of a chemical agent whether accidental or deliberate constitutes a chemical incident in the civil setting and a chemical attack in warfare. This chapter presents the overall management of civil chemical (HAZMAT) releases from the standpoint of the management of the incident. Early medical management of toxic trauma must be dynamically integrated with the management of the incident. An understanding of how chemical incidents are managed safely is an essential prerequisite for emergency medical personnel. Application of measures for detection, protection and decontamination must therefore precede any medical intervention. The stages of management of chemical incidents by responding emergency services are described in relation to HAZMAT hot, warm and cold zones. Some countries now deploy trained and protected emergency medical and paramedical personnel into the contaminated warm zone where they can provide essential early life support and organise safe evacuation of casualties to hospital emergency departments.

5.1 Introduction

Emergency medical personnel managing toxic trauma in hospitals may be involved in the incident itself either as part of the pre-hospital response teams, as is the case in France and other European countries, or because of the need to manage contaminated casualties who arrive at the emergency department without having been processed through a chemical incident management system (HAZMAT). Such contaminated casualties may pose a serious risk to the hospital personnel and their activities.

It is therefore important that medical responders understand all aspects of the potential hazards of the release of toxic chemicals. The management of chemical releases is usually done by specialist arms of the fire and rescue services and the police and involves considerable detail about the properties of the agents involved. However, there is a need for medical teams to be aware of the principles of management of chemical incidents, particularly in the provision of emergency life support within a contaminated area.

© Springer International Publishing Switzerland 2016
D.J. Baker, *Toxic Trauma*, DOI 10.1007/978-3-319-40916-0_5

5.2   Definitions

Since chemical incidents are so varied in nature, they are difficult to define. As a result, several definitions are used:

- The Public Health Service in England defines them as all incidents representing 'an acute event in which there is, or could be, exposure of the public to chemical substances which cause, or have the potential to cause, ill health'. All incidents with an off-site impact, as well as on-site incidents where members of the public are affected, are included in this definition and, for the purposes of the definition, hospital staff and emergency services personnel should be regarded as members of the public.
- The International Programme on Chemical Safety (a joint activity of the World Health Organization, the International Labour Organization and the United Nations Environment Programme) (IPCS 2010) provides the following three definitions:

  - **Chemical Incident** An uncontrolled release of a chemical from its containment that either threatens to or does expose people to a chemical hazard (WHO/IPCS 1999, Public Health and Chemical Incidents: Guidance for National and Regional Policy Makers in the Public/Environmental Health Roles). Such an incident could occur accidentally, for example a chemical spill, or deliberately, for example the use of sarin on a public transport system. In both cases, the release of the chemical or chemicals is usually obvious.
  - **Chemical Emergency** A chemical incident that has passed the control capability of one emergency service.
  - **Acute Public Health Chemical Incident** A public health chemical incident where the exposure dose is rising or is likely to rise rapidly and where rapid public health measures may limit the exposure.

Note that the IPCS definition above means a chemical incident that has passed the control capability of one emergency service and requires a joint response. For large-scale toxic releases, this is usually the case.

5.3   Identifying a Chemical Incident

The cause of a conventional major trauma incident is usually the violent release of energy, for example, from an explosion and fire or overwhelming environmental situations such as earthquakes or floods. In conventional incidents involving physical trauma, the consequences and the history and presentation of casualties are clearly linked to the event. However, major chemical releases may be less readily identifiable and the relationship with presenting casualties with toxic trauma less clear. There may be evidence of grouped casualties, but there may also be insidious presentation of sporadic casualties occurring without warning and only coincident symptoms or signs which at first may be unidentifiable. Chapter 4 covered the essential indicators of the possibility of a toxic release. In the multiagency management of a declared chemical incident, detailed information about the nature of the release and its onward consequences will be available from detection, identification and monitoring equipment carried by fire and some emergency medical services.

5.3.1   Controlling the Release and Transmission of a Toxic Hazard

Although mass chemical incidents are relatively unfamiliar, there are many analogies that will be familiar to emergency medical personnel from the management of conventional mass trauma. In incidents as different as multiple vehicle crash on a motorway or the detonation of a terrorist-improvised explosive device, the safety of responding emergency services has a high priority. The first stage in this is to establish a protective cordon around the incident site, which is controlled by the police. Within this cordon, rescue and life-support care is provided before casualties are evacuated to hospital care.

In chemical agent releases, the analogue to this protective cordon is determined by the fire services or HAZMAT specialists but is again enforced and controlled by the police who act under fire and rescue guidance about the hazards involved, based upon detection and identification procedures described earlier. The principal purpose of this cordon is to permit rescue and life support for casualties as early as possible but with an emphasis on protecting emergency responders becoming the next casualties from the toxic release.

In the HAZMAT system, there is a priority in establishing a hot zone, which is the area where direct contact and contamination from the released chemical takes place. It is the task of the fire and rescue services to remove casualties from this zone as soon as possible. Access to the hot zone is restricted to trained personnel, equipped with the appropriate quality of chemical protective clothing and, if necessary, self-contained breathing apparatus. If the nature of the released hazard has not been established, the fire service personnel usually enter the hot zone wearing level A protection with a self-contained breathing apparatus.

Immediately surrounding the hot zone of a chemical release is the warm zone. This too is contaminated but with the difference that the contamination is secondary from the hot zone, having been spread by persons exiting either rescuers and their equipment or on the clothing of contaminated casualties. It is in the warm zone that early decontamination of exposed persons takes place and triage, life-support and early antidote care for casualties. Rescuers exiting the warm zone must also undergo decontamination. Outside the warm zone is the cold zone which is regarded as being uncontaminated and where the advanced medical post, familiar from conventional physical disaster management, is situated. Here, re-triage and

Fig. 5.1 HAZMAT
organisation into zones

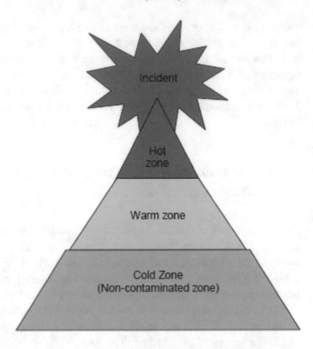

further stabilising medical care can be provided before casualties are transported to the hospital. Figure 5.1 shows the overall scheme of incident management following a toxic agent release. Box 5.1 lists the role of emergency medical responders at each stage of the HAZMAT chain.

Box 5.1 Role of the emergency medical responder at each stage of the HAZMAT management chain

- Hot zone: Usually none, but in some circumstances (such as entrapment) emergency care, may be needed

Warm zone

- Triage
- Immediate management

  – Life support and antidotes
  – Decontamination with continuing medical management

Cold zone

- Advanced medical post
- Re-triage
- Latency-dependent toxidromes
- Continuing life support
- Management of mixed injury

Transfer to hospital care

- Potential ED problems
- Contamination checks
- Continuing hazard for ED personnel

5.4 Important Points for Emergency Medical Personnel Responding to a Chemical Incident

5.4.1 Organisation

Chemical incidents are often complex in nature and may lead to a disproportionate amount of disruption compared to other types of incident. In addition, many different emergency and rescue services may become involved, along with other agencies and authorities. This interagency partnership is characteristic of the response to chemical incidents. As a result of these factors, collaboration and efficient communication with all the involved units is vital. Medical teams must work in collaboration with both the fire and rescue services who will establish the degree of hazard involved and the police who have the responsibility for maintaining the HAZMAT cordon and also investigating a potential crime scene if a terrorist toxic release is suspected. This may lead to a conflict of priorities between the police and emergency medical responders since the police will wish to preserve the chain of evidence which involves disturbing the site as little as possible.

5.4.2 Recognition, Reconnaissance and Reporting of a Chemical Incident

Essential features of the recognition of a chemical release were considered in the previous chapter. Application of these principles is essential to the continuing safe management of a chemical incident. In some cases, a responding emergency medical team may be the first on scene. In this situation, an important responsibility of those arriving first and who suspect a chemical release is to ensure that the appropriate help has been summoned.

5.4.3   Reconnaissance

It is also essential to pass on information about the exact location, type and severity of the release, hazards, the number of casualties present and access. The UK ambulance services use simple mnemonics to facilitate this task which are shown in Box 5.2.

Box 5.2 Mnemonics used by ambulance services for reporting a HAZMAT incident 'METHANE'

My call sign/major incident alert
Exact location
Type of incident
Hazards at the scene
Access
Number of casualties and severity
Emergency services present or required

'CHALETS'

Casualties, number and severity
Hazards, present and potential
Access and egress
Location—exact
Emergency services—present or required
Type of incident
Safety

5.4.4   Approaching the Incident: Key Actions

1. If called to a potential chemical scene, the approach should be cautious, uphill and upwind from the release.
2. On arrival, all medical staff should identify the officer in charge of the incident—the incident commander (this will usually be a senior fire or police officer), the incident command centre if it is already set up. The presence of each worker and any special skills, equipment or knowledge that they have can then be logged. Preparation should be made for the use of PPE at this time (see Chap. 4). Respiratory protection is the most important aspect of this and respirators should be kept close by to allow rapid donning if the situation deteriorates and there is immediate airborne contamination (e.g. from a change in wind direction).
3. At this time, emergency responders will be given a precise role, e.g. medical commander, hazard advisor or triage officer. It is important to keep to this allocated role so that duplication and confusion are minimised. As with the

management of mass disasters involving physical trauma, recognition of the medical personnel involved in the response and their duties (doctor, nurse, paramedic) is important. Wearing high-visibility identification jackets is now a standard procedure.

4. Once the overall scene has been assessed by the incident commander, implementation of any local pre-agreed on- or off-site plans or major incident policies can be instituted.

5. One of the main difficulties of a chemical incident is obtaining rapid information on the identity of the chemical or mix of chemicals involved and their health hazards. Disseminating this information is vital and allows medical management to proceed on an adequately informed basis. Evidence of the nature of the released chemical will come from the detection equipment deployed by the fire and special ambulance services and also from the primary assessment of the signs and symptoms of casualties to try and identify characteristic toxidromes. These are considered in Chap. 6.

5.5 Clinical Operations Within a Chemical Incident

Details about the medical management of toxic trauma in both the pre-hospital and hospital settings are given in Chap. 8. Within the context of chemical incident management, the following are the key points in the provision of emergency care:

1. The number of emergency personnel involved in the management of contaminated casualties should be kept to the minimum in order to contain any potential risks of secondary contamination. Emergency medical responders must always be alert to the dangers of the spread of contamination throughout all stages of resuscitation and treatment of casualties.

2. Circumstances, weather conditions and information on contamination can all change, so it is vital to stay in communication with the incident control unit. Similarly, it is also important to be aware that unusual chemicals or mixtures of agents may have been released which can lead to the development of unpredictable or unexpected toxic effects. The importance of latency of signs and symptoms in presenting casualties must always be remembered.

3. One of the main aims of management of contaminated casualties is for them to be managed as close to the scene as feasible without compromising patient care or putting responders at undue risk. This minimises the potential spread of contamination whilst also allowing early resuscitation. Combined with decontamination, this approach optimises the chances for recovery of casualties. It is also important to remember that casualties of a chemical incident may also have sustained physical trauma as either a primary or secondary feature. Many national emergency services now plan for essential advanced life support to be provided in the warm zone, together with resuscitation, and have trained special paramedical and medical teams for this purpose.

5.6   Triage

Triage of casualties following any disaster is an essential procedure to use the available medical resources to provide the greatest benefit to the greatest number of injured. Triage was originally introduced by Baron Larrey during the Napoleonic Wars (see Chap. 2). An overall modern triage scheme for mass casualties with physical trauma is as follows:

1. *Immediate* (*P1*): casualties who require life-saving care within a short time, when that care is available and of short duration.
2. *Delayed* (*P2*): casualties with severe injuries who are in need of major or prolonged surgery or other care and who will require hospitalisation, but delay of this care will not adversely affect the outcome of the injury.
3. *Minimal* (*P3*): casualties who have minor injuries, can be helped by non-physician medical personnel and will not be evacuated to hospital.
4. *Expectant* (*P4*): casualties with severe life-threatening injuries who would not survive with optimal medical care, or casualties whose injuries are so severe that their chance of survival does not justify expenditure of resources.

A modification of this system to the management of toxic trauma is as follows:

T1: resuscitation required *during decontamination* in a stretcher facility
T2: treatment may be delayed until after decontamination in a stretcher facility
T3: minor injuries, may walk unaided to an ambulant decontamination facility
T4: expectant

In the HAZMAT context, T4 is usually taken to mean a casualty who is not breathing despite having an open airway. However, as will be discussed in the next chapter in this situation, respiratory failure may not yet have produced the end stage secondary cardiac arrest which is the terminal event in toxic trauma. The use of T4 in chemical incidents remains controversial. Airway and ventilatory support should be provided whilst the cardiac status is being assessed. This will depend on the conditions applied and the number of casualties being treated.

If a three-zone HAZMAT response is necessary, initial triage should be carried out in the warm zone by the most senior physician or paramedical person available. If this is not possible, primary triage should be carried out immediately after leaving the warm zone in the advanced medical post. In toxic trauma, frequent re-triage is necessary due to developing conditions as a result of latency.

Further discussion of triage with examples of casualties from specific toxic agents in each class will be found in Chap. 8

5.7 Decontamination in the Warm Zone

The importance of decontamination to reduce exposure and secondary transmission of a toxic hazard was discussed in Chap. 4. In any toxic release, the need for decontamination depends on the persistency of the released toxic agent. However, even if an agent is persistent, not all persons in or near a release zone will require decontamination. Persons held in the warm zone of the cordon where a persistent agent has been used may be classed as follows:

1. Uninjured and non-contaminated
2. Toxic trauma and contaminated
3. Injured and non-contaminated (from the effects of physical trauma)
4. Both physical and toxic trauma with contamination

The use of detection and monitoring equipment will determine the classes of patient and different flow lines out of the warm zone can be established.

Figures 5.2 and 5.3 show diagrammatically the warm zone flow lines used by the French emergency medical service.

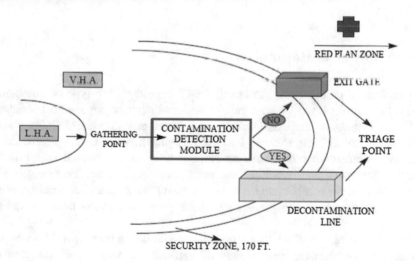

Fig. 5.2 HAZMAT zone arrangement (Plan Rouge) used by the French fire and rescue service (*LHA* liquid hazard (hot) zone; *VHA* vapour hazard (warm) zone). Triage is conducted (1) to detect contamination (2) for medical status in the triage point or the AMP. Later modifications of the plan allow for the provision of early life support by emergency medical personnel when required inside the warm zone (figure reproduced by courtesy of SAMU de Paris)

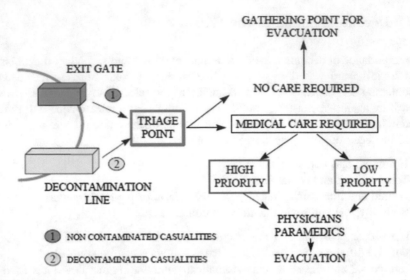

Fig. 5.3 Plan Piratox (modified red plan) management of toxic trauma casualties in France. In the French emergency medical service (SAMU), emergencies are classified as either absolute or relative. The decision is based upon the medical experience (figure reproduced by courtesy of SAMU de Paris)

5.8 Transfer to Hospital

The transfer of casualties to the hospital will depend on the type of emergency medical service deployed. Some countries such as France deploy medical personnel with the ambulance response teams, and these can provide definitive early life-support and antidote treatment whilst delaying transfer. Other paramedically operated ambulance services have an early transfer to the hospital as a priority, delaying treatment until reaching the emergency department. Factors affecting transfer include the number and severity of contaminated casualties, location of the incident, weather conditions, distance to the appropriate medical facilities and the resources available.

Vehicles taking casualties to the hospital should take a route that does not pass through any contaminated areas or plumes. Vehicles used to transport contaminated casualties should be separated from other vehicles and used only for the incident. All equipment and devices used during the incident should be kept together in order to facilitate comprehensive decontamination at the end of the incident. Past experience has shown that there can be secondary contamination from the use of contaminated equipment, clothing or vehicles.

Advance warning for any receiving hospitals is essential so that emergency procedures can be implemented. It is important to note that casualties may have self-evacuated and may arrive at the hospital or the emergency department without warning. Consequently, prompt action is always necessary. Information is needed

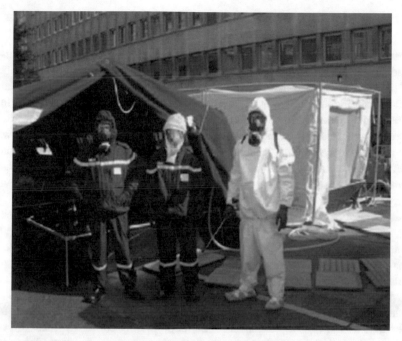

Fig. 5.4 Reception and decontamination facilities for toxic trauma casualties at a French hospital designated for the reception of chemical casualties. Access to the hospital is through one specific entrance for contaminated casualties. The emergency physicians are wearing level C protection with filtration respirators stored at the hospital (photograph courtesy of SAMU de Paris)

as to whether casualties have been decontaminated at the scene or whether decontamination will be needed at the hospital. A separate area for ambulances should be allocated so that they can be decontaminated after the incident. Figure 5.4 shows a typical hospital decontamination/casualty reception.

5.9   Incident Documentation

Clear documentation of a chemical incident is essential, not only for safe management of casualties but also as a record that may be required legally for any subsequent inquiry that may be held. Essential data such as the date and time of the release should be recorded as well as the source of the first reports. Although writing detailed notes is not always possible during the management stages of an incident, a definitive record should be completed as soon as possible afterwards. It should be accurate, clear and informative to be of use for debriefing purposes.

5.10   Debriefing and Feedback

Chemical agent releases usually occur without warning and often require the use of already overstretched resources. Medical professionals may be concerned about the effectiveness of the response. A 'hot debrief' as the incident ends can often identify problems not identified by advanced emergency planning and allow an opportunity for early remediation. Most importantly, concerns may exist about the hazard and any risk to workers that might have arisen during the response. It is essential where such risks are identified that medical help is sought. This help may include a proper medical assessment and even triage along with other casualties, which may lead to referral to hospital, GP or occupational health department depending on the severity of any illness.

A 'hot debrief' also allows individuals concerned in the response to express any anxieties or fears over their ability to respond. For instance, it may highlight problems in identification of the hazard. Further investigation may be required by other collaborating agencies or organisations. Planned interagency debriefing helps to identify communication issues and clarify roles and responsibilities. It also allows an appropriate team to continue any longer-term investigation into an incident. It is vital that all those who have played a part in the response to an incident make the time to participate in the appropriate debriefing process in order to ensure an ability to contribute more effectively next time, and that plans can be improved. Good documentation facilitates debriefing and feedback.

5.11   Planning for Toxic Incidents

Chemical incident planning should be integrated into standard hospital disaster plans and should have the direct involvement of emergency medical staff who will be expected to receive casualties with toxic trauma.

Planning involves the following four stages:

- Prevention
- Preparedness
- Response
- Recovery

Prevention This section of the plan allows for improved incident documentation to identify and provide strategies to reduce incidents. It should also include hazard control, surveillance and identification of incidents, and the development of strategies to reduce hazards, along with education.

Preparedness Plans for chemical incidents should include active preparation in a number of areas, e.g. patient decontamination. Health and safety issues of responders and personal protective clothing provision should be considered and documented by availability and location. Training in the use of these plans and specific aspects, such as when to wear and how useful is personal protective clothing, is essential.

Response Within the plans should be included documentation needed during the response, including incident logs, checklists and material related to specific sampling, public safety and clean-up measures.

Recovery This deals with reviewing the incident and auditing the response, legal proceedings and feedback on processes (lessons learned). It can be invaluable in determining any risk to the responders and in improving plans for the future. Clinicians should be directly involved with this process to provide information about the effectiveness of the hospital response and identify potential weak points.

5.12   New Directions in the Management of Toxic Trauma: An Example Developed by the International Committee of the Red Cross and Red Crescent

5.12.1   Introduction

This chapter has so far considered the conventional approaches to the management of casualties of toxic trauma as part of existing HAZMAT protocols. Despite the fact that there is increasing interest in providing early medical care in a contaminated area, there are still wide divergences between the medical management of chemical incidents and that of other disasters where the casualties produced suffer from conventional trauma.

There is a requirement to integrate management of casualties from toxic trauma into existing patterns of casualty management elsewhere. In particular, there is no direct equivalent with the basic and advanced life support which is defined in systems such as basic life support (BLS), advanced life support (ALS) and basic trauma life support (BTLS™) and advanced trauma life support (ATLS™). There has been a feeling for many years that the general public can play no part in the early stages of a chemical incident, and little has been done to make provision for simple training and the provision of equipment that could reduce casualties (particularly from inhalational injury) shortly after a toxic agent release. This is in marked contrast to the situation shortly before and during the Second World War when there was a constant fear of mass civilian gas attacks from the air which was countered by programmes of civil defence awareness on both sides and particularly by the mass issue of gas masks. Since that time, with the threat of aerial gas attack receding, civil training and equipment for response to a chemical attack has become practically non-existent in many countries (with the exception of the Middle East where the threat of civil chemical exposure has remained since the 1980s).

There is a requirement, therefore, for improved civilian training and training of medical responders to be able to counter chemical agent release at both a basic and advanced level. In 2012, the International Committee of the Red Cross and Red Crescent (ICRC) launched a new initiative to define competences in response to chemical agent release (and also for biological and radiological agent release) and to start suitable training programmes. This initiative is based upon the specific requirements for their own field medical teams and other personnel who may be caught in chemical incidents as a result of their being present to provide humanitarian assistance in disaster and civil conflicts.

5.12.2 Objectives and Rationale of Chemical Agent Management Within the International Committee of the Red Cross and Red Crescent Societies

The programme set up by the ICRC covered possible casualties from exposure to nuclear, biological, radiological (radioisotope) and chemical agents. The discussion here focuses only on chemical agents causing toxic trauma.

Overall, the objectives of the ICRC initiative were to:

1. define levels at which protection and medical care could be provided
2. start a programme of training that would take a fresh approach to chemical casualty management across the entire civil spectrum to improve medical outcome.

The ICRC work started in 2009 because of the publication of a global risk assessment on the use of chemical, biological, radiological and nuclear (CBRN) weapons and the observation at the time that an international response to assist the victims was not feasible. Thus, the decision was made by ICRC to provide specific training and equipping for its field teams to provide a self-contained response. It was recognised that the medical assistance required relates to a field of medicine where real experience is scarce but that necessary responses can be based on clinical analogy from accidental exposures and from other clinical conditions.

Since the start of the Red Cross initiative, world events have shown its relevance already in two prominent chemical release contexts: (1) in relation to the concerns about the existence of, access to and the potential use of chemical weapons in Libya and the resulting risk to the ICRC staff following the outbreak of hostilities in February 2011; and (2) in relation to the use of chemical weapons in the civil conflict in Damascus since 2013 (see Chap. 10).

5.12.3 Specific Elements of the ICRC Chemical Response Initiative

Three main objectives of the new initiative were identified in the following order priority:

- Health, safety and security of staff
- Continuation of ICRC presence and humanitarian operations
- Assistance to victims whether directly affected (e.g. exposed to toxic agents) or indirectly affected (e.g. displaced by the event)

This targeted approach was conceived by an organisation that has a mandate to provide impartial medical care in a wide range of circumstances. It provides a model for other organisations (such as medical non-governmental organisations) who may be faced with similar problems of unexpected exposure to toxic chemical agent release whilst working in conflict zones.

5.12.3.1 Agent-Specific Considerations

In general terms, the ICRC initiative recognised that a chemical agent's toxicity and latency determine the health impact on a person who has been exposed to an agent, whereas persistency and the physical form of the agent determine the management of a response in a potentially contaminated environment (see Chap. 3) From this, it was evident that potentially life-saving medical assistance at field level has to focus on agents with high toxicity and short latency which constitutes a range of chemical agents and toxins.

5.12.3.2 Medical Assistance as Part of the ICRC Chemical Response Capacity

The Red Cross and Red Crescent have recognised that when mounting an operational response to a chemical release, the risk against which potential benefit must be balanced depends not only on the nature and extent of release and dispersal of the agent but also on the availability and effectiveness of three core capacities. These are as follows:

- Individual or collective protection against the agent in question
- Management of exposure to and contamination by the agent in question (including detection and monitoring, decontamination and waste management)
- Medical care for contaminated or potentially contaminated people

With regard to medical assistance, this entails specifying what care needs to be available at and away from the site of release of the agent, both in support of ICRC staff and operations and for assisting victims of the event.

5.12.3.3 ICRC-Defined Levels of Care for Toxic Trauma

In general, management of hazardous material release protocols exists for the management of people suffering toxic trauma inside a contaminated area by specially equipped and trained paramedical and medical teams. In the HAZMAT model, medical care is provided following a release of a hazardous material and assumes that three zones of operation (hot, warm and cold) can be established quickly.

This approach, however, is based on certain assumptions including that:

- The event requires a coordinated post-release response.
- There is a single release at a known location and with determinable contamination level.
- There is the means for localised containment of the released agents (by, e.g., preventing contaminated people from leaving the area).
- The responders have the authority to respond to the event.
- In the humanitarian aid scenarios most likely to be encountered by the ICRC, these assumptions cannot be necessarily be made. In general, the ICRC has to be prepared to respond:
- To confirmed, threatened and alleged release of CBRN agents (pre- and/or post-release response)
- To unconfirmed release points (single or multiple, local or widespread)
- Where contamination levels are unknown
- Where localised containment is absent or has failed (resulting in, e.g., contaminated people presenting at other health facilities)
- In contexts of unclear existing response capacities and authority
- Where there is a lack of appropriate medical personnel and material (including hospital facilities)

Integral to the conventional approach to chemical agent casualty management is that any medical assistance will be provided by appropriately trained medical professionals. In contrast, the approach proposed by the ICRC states that not only is medical care possible in a contaminated or potentially contaminated environment but also that non-medical emergency responders could provide some effective first aid.

Two levels of care have therefore been proposed:

1. Basic life support for toxic trauma provided by non-medical responders who are present at or near the site of the chemical release. This is the chemical equivalent of basic life and trauma support or 'first aid'
2. Advanced life support for toxic trauma provided by medical responders who are trained in ALS and ATLS[TM] protocols and who are able to respond safely within a contaminated zone

5.12.3.4   Basic Care for Casualties with Toxic Trauma

It is recognised that a basic response to chemical agent release provided by trained non-medical persons with little or no medical equipment can be effective as a primary response. This basic life support and basic trauma life support constitute 'first aid'. To date, the notion of applying first aid to people suffering toxic trauma in a contaminated or potentially contaminated environment has not been widely explored. Measures that could be employed include minimising further exposure to a toxic agent and basic gestures to ensure airway patency such as placing an unconscious patient in a lateral position. Giving a clear and structured report of the incident is also an important part of any primary response. The scope of the basic toxic trauma life support level is shown in Box 5.3.

Box 5.3 International Red Cross basic measures for the management of toxic trauma (2012)

Chemical basic (first aid) measures for the management of toxic trauma can be provided by non-medical personnel with basic training and access to no or only basic medical equipment. In addition to basic life support and trauma management skills, additional features required are as follows:

- A basic understanding of the differences between the classes of agents with high toxicity and short transmissibility (notably classical chemical warfare agents) and recognition of the corresponding toxidromes
- Training in the use of auto-injectors in the event of exposure to a nerve agent
- The capability to provide this basic life support in a potentially contaminated environment, i.e. whilst wearing protective equipment

---

5.12.3.5   Field-level (Advanced) Medical Assistance for Toxic Trauma

Specific measures have been identified in developing a field-level medical assistance component. This involves defining the skills, equipment and information necessary to recognise the most likely toxidromes and treat the affected person accordingly whilst optimising the protection of the responder from exposure to the agent responsible for the toxic trauma.

The overall objective is patient survival and stabilisation. The ICRC foresees field-level medical assistance in a contaminated or potentially contaminated environment bringing together:

- The recognition that the principles of both advanced and basic life support (maintaining the airway, supporting ventilation, arresting haemorrhage and supporting circulation) can also be applied to people suffering acute life-threatening effects of CBRN agents, supported by specific antidotes if necessary.
- The recognition that the treatment of toxic trauma based on these principles is only needed and would only be effective for people affected by chemical agents with high toxicity and short latency.
- The recognition that treatment of conventional or toxic trauma in potential toxic environments requires access to and use of appropriate personnel protective equipment.
- The assumption that these measures would have potential benefit whether or not there is access to hospital care.

The scope of the advanced toxic trauma response level is shown in Box 5.4.

Box 5.4 International Red Cross advanced (field medical care) measures for the management of toxic trauma (2012)

Chemical advanced (field medical care) measures for the management of toxic trauma can be provided by suitably equipped medical professionals who, as part of their normal professional activities, manage patients suffering cardiorespiratory arrest and in particular are familiar with airway management including endotracheal intubation (i.e. anaesthetists, emergency room physicians and paramedics). The training and equipment must be suitable for providing advanced life support whether or not patients can reach hospital care. In addition to advanced life support and trauma management skills, additional features required are as follows:

- A thorough understanding of the classes of agents with high toxicity and short transmissibility (notably classical chemical warfare agents) and recognition of the corresponding toxidromes
- A broad understanding of other chemical, biological, radiological and nuclear (CBRN) agents;
- Training in the use of specific antidotes in the event of exposure to CBRN agents;
- The capability to provide this advanced life support in a potentially contaminated environment, i.e. whilst wearing protective equipment.

Psychological assessment and support skills are also important at this level of care, due to the inherent fear of chemical agents which could result in the 'worried well' overloading any medical capacity to the detriment of casualties who have defined somatic injury.

Apart from providing life-saving and other early treatment measures, the first aid and field medical care skill levels are designed to stabilise the seriously ill patients for evacuation for hospital care, i.e. emergency and intensive care at a fully

Table 5.1 ICRC-defined medical skills required for basic and advanced care of toxic trauma

	Toxic chemical agent release recognition	Diagnosis	Airway	Ventilation	Circulation	Investigation/Monitoring/Specific care	Antidotes and supportive therapy	Medical decontamination	Communications
First aid	Sensory indicators (e.g. smell, visual observations)	General toxidrome recognition, if possible (class of agent)	Note[c]	Note[c]	Note[c]	Note[c]	Combopen[e]	Emergency decontamination (e.g. RSDL, eye irrigation)	Call for help
	Unusual clusters of illnesses	Triage (first aid level)	BLS procedures	Portable gas-powered ventilation via mask and Guedel airway or bag-valve device with filter	BLS level management of haemorrhage control	Patient conscious level[d]	Salbutamol		Situation report[f]
	Other indicators (e.g. intelligence, threats)[a]		Lateral position			Conventional physical and psychological trauma treatment (equivalent BTLS)			
	DIM[b] information		Chin lift						
			Suction						
			Guedel airway						
Field medical care	Agent class recognition	Specific toxidrome recognition	As for BLS plus ALS procedures	Oxygen free-flow or demand delivery system	IV or IO access	Detailed patient conscious level	Salbutamol	Decontamination (assisted ambulant/non-ambulant) for persistent agents	To hospital care level and on-site control
	DIM information	Clinical examination/evaluation	Laryngeal mask airway	Bag-valve ventilation (with filter)		Pulse oximetry	Atropine		Liaison with emergency services
		Triage, re - evaluation and decontamination	Endotracheal tube (intubation)	Portable gas-powered ventilation (with filter)		End-tidal CO_2	Oximes		

(continued)

Table 5.1 (continued)

Toxic chemical agent release recognition	Diagnosis	Airway	Ventilation	Circulation	Investigation/Monitoring/Specific care	Antidotes and supportive therapy	Medical decontamination	Communications
					Respiratory rate and pattern (scale of respiratory failure)	Inhaled and systemic steroids		
					Non-invasive blood pressure	Anti-CN agents		
					Electrocardiogram	Antibiotics		
					Simple blood count (Hb and white cell)	Potassium iodide		
					Conventional physical and psychological trauma treatment (equivalent ATLS) and care for pre-existing medical conditions			

[a] e.g. standard triggers for emergency personnel in detecting a CBRN event (STEP 1, 2, 3)

[b] LM detection/identification/monitoring

[c] S= International Liaison Committee on Resuscitation Guidelines on Basic Life Support (2010)

[d] e.g. simple consciousness level assessment by AVPU scale: Alert and responding normally, Voice response, Painful stimuli response, Unresponsive

[e] Requires agreed and approved administration rules (e.g. PGD)

[f] e.g. CHALETS reporting: Casualties (number and severity), Hazards (identified, present and potential), Location (exact position of the release), Emergency services (present, required?), Type of event (signs indicating nuclear, radiological, biological or chemical)

equipped non-contaminated hospital. Such facilities are present in urban general and university hospitals or military facilities but may be scarce in many of the contexts in which the ICRC works. In this situation, if there is a real need, time and resources, hospital care facilities could be improvised (e.g. by extended CBRN field medical care resources) or set up by bringing in considerable specialised resources. Otherwise, this level of care may only be made available by sophisticated medical air-evacuation capacities.

5.12.3.6 Specific Basic and Advanced Skills for the Management of Toxic Trauma

The ICRC toxic trauma care measures have defined the specific paramedical and medical skills required at both the basic and advanced levels. These are summarised in Table 5.1.

The recent Red Cross initiative for management of casualties from toxic trauma and also from exposure to biological and radiological agents (which are outside the scope of this discussion) provided a concrete example of the integration of medical management of toxic in the realm of conventional trauma. It builds upon existing emergency management skills in areas that are relatively familiar into an area where they are often not. Importantly, the definition of both basic and advanced life-support measures following a toxic agent release in their model provides an example that could be applied in other settings to allow (1) the general public to minimise the effects of chemical releases and apply simple measures that will reduce harm and (2) emergency medical responders to apply their existing knowledge in reducing morbidity and mortality from what is likely to be an unfamiliar and unexpected event.

5.13 Conclusions

An understanding of chemical incident management and the way casualties are managed at the point of release and through to the hospital emergency room is essential for all emergency medical personnel. Standard HAZMAT procedures manage toxic releases by a series of protected zones which are designed to minimise onward transmission of toxic hazards. Nevertheless, the arrival of contaminated casualties at a hospital occurred in previous HAZMAT incidents, and emergency departments should have measures in place to deal with them safely by suitably trained and equipped staff. Planning for toxic agent release should be an integral part of all hospital disaster responses.

Further Reading

Advanced Life Support Group (2002) Major incident medical management and support: the practical approach, 2nd edn. BMJ Publishing, London

Baker DJ (2007) The management of casualties following toxic agent release: the approach adopted in France. In: Marrs TC, Maynard RL, Sidell FR (eds) Chemical warfare agents: toxicology and treatment. Wiley, Chichester, pp 261–276 (Chap. 12)

Briggs SM, Brinsfiled KH (2003) Advanced disaster medical response manual for providers. Harvard Medical International Inc, ISBN 0-9723772-0–4

Department of Health (2005) The NHS emergency planning guidance 2005. www.dh.gov.uk. Accessed 8 June 2013

Fisher J, Morgan-Jones D, Murray V, Davies G (1999) Chemical incident management for accident and emergency physicians. The Stationery Office, London

Heptonstall J, Gent N (2006) CRBN incidents: clinical management and health protection. Health Protection Agency, London. ISBN: 0901144703. http://www.hpa.org.uk/web/HPAwebFile/HPAweb_C/1194947377166. Accessed 6 June 2013

International Programme on Chemical Safety (WHO/ILO/UNEP) (2010) Key definitions. http://www.who.int/ipcs/emergencies/definitions/en/index.html. Accessed 11 April 2013

Jane's Mass Casualty Handbook: prehospital (2003) Jane' Information Group, Coulsdon, Surrey, UK

Jane's Chem—Bio Handbook. 2nd edition (2003) Jane' Information Group, Coulsdon, Surrey, UK

Malich G, Coupland R, Donelly S, Baker D (2012) A proposal for field—level medical assistance in an international humanitarian response to chemical, biological, radiological or nuclear events. Emerg Med J 30:804–808. doi:10.1136/emermed-2012-201915

Murray VSG, Baker DJ (2011) Chemical incidents. In: Practical prehospital care: the principles and practice of immediate care, Chap. 49. Churchill Livingstone, Elsevier, London, pp 503–513

WHO/IPCS (1999) Public health and chemical incidents: guidance for national and regional policy makers in the public/environmental health roles. http://www.who.int/ipcs/publications/en/Public_Health_Management.pdf. Accessed 11 April 2013

Chapter 6
The Pathophysiology of Toxic Trauma

Abstract The mechanisms and mediators of physical trauma have been intensively studied over the past three decades and have led to a better understanding of the rational management of injury both in the immediate care and longer-term intensive care phases. Equally, there has been study of the mechanisms of toxic trauma which converge with those found in physical trauma in conditions such as the acute respiratory distress syndrome and multiple organ dysfunction. This chapter considers the effects of exposure to toxic substances in terms of their effects on target organs of the various systems of the body. An understanding of the mechanisms involved in the pathophysiology of toxic trauma is essential to the rational clinical management of casualties who have been exposed to toxic chemical agents, both in the shorter and longer term. In recent years, there has been intense research into the mechanisms of toxic trauma, particularly to the respiratory and nervous systems, and there is a wealth of detailed information available in the literature. Here, we consider the essentials which have relevance to practical clinical management.

6.1 Introduction

The past three decades have seen a great interest in the mechanisms and management of conventional physical trauma. This has been accompanied by a detailed understanding of the final pathways of the effects of trauma through shock and its effects on the organs of the body which has improved management. In parallel with this approach, this chapter considers the effects of exposure to toxic substances in terms of their effects on target organs of the various systems of the body. An understanding of the pathophysiology of these exposures is essential to being able to assess, diagnose and manage patients who have been subjected to toxic trauma. In the final stages of damage to target organs and somatic systems, there are pathways of damage such as acute respiratory distress syndrome that are common to both physical and toxic trauma.

© Springer International Publishing Switzerland 2016
D.J. Baker, *Toxic Trauma*, DOI 10.1007/978-3-319-40916-0_6

6.2   Targets for Toxic Trauma

A systemic, target organ-based approach used in physical trauma may also be adopted for patients exposed to toxic substances. These may have effects on one or several systems of the body and give rise to the presenting signs and symptoms of toxic trauma. The body systems that can be affected by toxic agents which will be considered are shown in Box 6.1.

Box 6.1 Somatic systems affected by toxic agents

Central nervous system
Peripheral nervous system
Respiratory system
Heart and central vascular system
Alimentary system
Urogenital system
Haemopoietic system

Overall, different systems are at risk depending on the route of toxic exposure. More than one system may be affected by a toxic exposure. As noted earlier, there may be both acute and chronic effects. The acute effects may be life-threatening in a short space of time. Toxic trauma concerns the immediate effects of exposure to high concentrations of toxic substances which may have occurred accidentally or deliberately. It should be distinguished from the effects of long-term exposure to low concentrations of toxic agents, although there are mechanisms of damage which are common to both types of exposure.

6.3   Toxic Trauma to the Nervous System

Both the central and peripheral nervous systems are made up of neurones that are linked to each other by chemical transmitters at synapses. Synaptic junctions serve to ensure the transmission of electrical nerve impulses from the brain to the organs controlled by the nerve pathway by achieving an amplification of the signal through chemical means. An understanding of the essential pharmacology of the nervous system is the first stage in understanding the effects of toxic substances at the synaptic level.

Equally, toxic agents both natural and man-made can act directly on the nerves themselves causing a failure in transmission, as in the case of many toxins which cause disruption of the ionic pump which controls the passage of the all-important sodium ions across the nerve membrane to ensure the passage of the nerve impulse.

6.3.1   The Function of the Cholinergic Nervous System

The cholinergic nervous system is a network of neurones spread through both the central and peripheral nervous systems which are characterised by synapses. Transmission of signals within the network is electrical except at the synapses where acetylcholine (ACh) is released to carry the impulses across a small gap to the next neurone or to an effector organ. It is ACh which gives the cholinergic nervous system its name. ACh is only one of the many chemical transmitters in the nervous system, whose function is to act as amplifying relay stations for the nerve impulses from the brain.

A great deal is known about ACh and the cholinergic nervous system. Detailed accounts of the physiology and pharmacology are beyond the scope of this chapter. Here, we concentrate on the essential function of ACh and cholinergic synapses from the standpoint of how transmission can be interrupted by toxic causes.

6.3.1.1   Synapses

Synapses are highly specialised gaps in the neural network. The arrival of a nerve impulse at the end of a neurone (the nerve terminal) releases ACh which diffuses across the small gap that comprises the synapse to the beginning of another neuron on the other side. Here, ACh combines with special receptors inducing another electric signal which is either transmitted towards another neurone or causes an effect on an adjacent organ such as a muscle fibre. Having completed the generation of a postsynaptic electric impulse, the ACh is quickly removed by the enzyme acetylcholinesterase which converts it back into choline and acetic acid which are taken up and reused in the nerve terminal. There are thus three key processes in cholinergic synaptic transmission: release of ACh, attachment of ACh to postsynaptic receptors, generating a new electrical signal and rapid enzymatic destruction of the transmitter which can then be reused. We shall see that each of these processes can be affected by toxic agents leading to a breakdown in cholinergic transmission with serious multi-organ toxic trauma.

6.3.1.2   Classification of Cholinergic Synapses

The basic structure of a synapse and the mechanism of cholinergic transmission are shown in Fig. 6.1. Within the cholinergic system, there are several different types of synapses which lead to different functions within both the autonomic and voluntary nervous systems. Shortly after the discovery by Otto Loewi in 1921 (Box 6.2) of ACh, it was found that there were two classes of synapses, termed muscarinic and

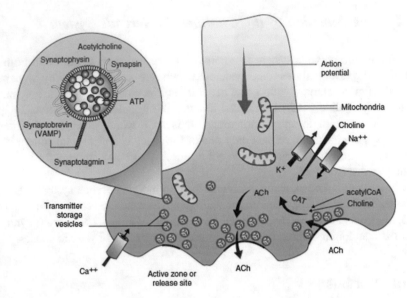

Fig. 6.1 The working of a chemical synapse, the motor nerve ending, including some of the apparatus for transmitter synthesis. The large, intracellular structures are mitochondria. Acetylcholine, synthesised from choline and acetate by acetyl coenzyme A, is transported into coated vesicles, which are moved to release sites. A presynaptic action potential, which triggers calcium influx through specialised proteins (Ca^{2+} channels), causes the vesicles to fuse with the membrane and discharge transmitter. Membrane from the vesicle is retracted from the nerve membrane and recycled. Each vesicle can undergo various degrees of release of content—from incomplete to complete. The transmitters inactivated by diffusion catabolism or reuptake. The *inset* provides a magnified view of a synaptic vesicle. Quanta of acetylcholine together with ATP are stored in the vesicle and covered by vesicle membrane protein. Synaptophysin is a vesicle membrane component glycoprotein. Synaptotagmin is the vesicle's calcium sensor. Phosphorylation of another membrane protein, synapsin, facilitates vesicular trafficking to the release site. Synaptobrevin (VAMP) is a SNARE protein, involved in attaching the vesicle to the release site. *ACh* acetylcholine, *acetyl CoA* acetyl coenzyme A, *CAT* choline acetyltransferase (from Martyn 2005, p 861; copyright Elsevier)

nicotinic. These names arose because transmission within the two types of synapse could be simulated in the laboratory by the use of two alkaloids muscarine and nicotine which acted on the synapses as false transmitters. Today, we know that there are many subclasses of muscarinic and nicotinic receptors but the original classification is still of value in understanding the clinical effects of toxic substances.

Box 6.2 Otto Loewi and the discovery of the actions of acetylcholine

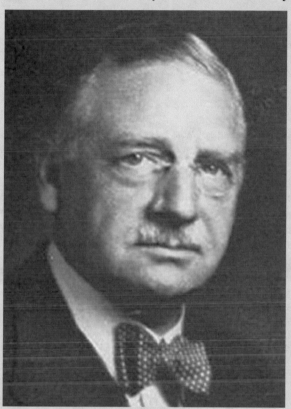

(*Source* Wikimedia Commons http://commons.wikimedia.org/wiki/File:Otto_Loewi_nobel.jpg)

Otto Loewi (1873–1961)

Otto Loewi was a distinguished German pharmacologist working in the earlier part of the twentieth century. He developed the concept of the chemical transmitter in a synapse, which had first been proposed in the late nineteenth century by the Frenchman Alfred Vulpian, (a pupil of Claude Bernard) in relation to the neuromuscular junction.

Loewi's most famous experiment, published in 1921, addressed the question of whether transmission at a synapse was chemical or electrical. He dissected out of frogs two beating hearts: one with the vagus nerve (the parasympathetic control) attached and the other detached from its nerve supply. Both hearts were bathed in Ringer's lactate solution in separate containers. By electrically stimulating the vagus nerve, Loewi made the first heartbeat slower. Then, Loewi took some of the liquid bathing the first heart and applied it to the second heart. The application of the liquid made the second heart also beat slower, proving that some soluble substance released by the vagus nerve was controlling the heart rate. The released chemical transmitter was later identified as acetylcholine.

Loewi went on to characterise the synapses of the autonomic nervous system as nicotinic or muscarinic (where acetylcholine mimics the action of nicotine or muscarine when directly applied to the synapse). This classification exists to the present day and has been developed to include subclasses of receptor.

For his work on chemical transmission, Loewi was awarded a Nobel Prize, jointly with the English pharmacologist Henry Dale in 1936.

Loewi was Jewish and had to move to the USA in 1940 where he continued his research. He died in New York City on Christmas Day, 1961.

Muscarinic receptors are found in both the brain and the peripheral nervous system. In the latter, they are within the autonomic (involuntary) nervous system where they control functions within the respiratory, cardiac, alimentary and urogenital systems. This is important in understanding the toxidromes (characteristic collections of signs and symptoms) which arise after toxic exposure. In the central nervous system (CNS), the muscarinic receptors are present in high proportions within several difference subtypes which are listed in Box 6.3.

Box 6.3 Muscarinic receptors

Many different subclasses of muscarinic receptor have been identified experimentally.

The simplest classification describes three types:

Muscarinic M1: located in CNS neurones, sympathetic postganglionic neurones and some presynaptic sites (e.g. neuromuscular junction, controlling the release of ACh).

Muscarinic M2: located in the myocardium, smooth muscle and some presynaptic sites.

Muscarinic M3: located in exocrine glands and ocular, gastrointestinal and urogenital smooth muscle and vascular endothelium.

In the peripheral autonomic nervous system, muscarinic synapses are found within the parasympathetic nervous system and give rise to actions which are the opposite of the protective, fight-or-flight responses of the sympathetic nervous system. Such well-known actions include slowing of the heart through the vagus nerve and contraction of the bowel. A simplified diagram of the parasympathetic nervous system and the organs it controls is shown in Fig. 6.2.

Nicotinic cholinergic receptors are also found in the autonomic nervous system where they act as an intermediary synapse in the sympathetic nervous system. Here, the final chemical transmitter is noradrenaline whose release gives rise to actions on

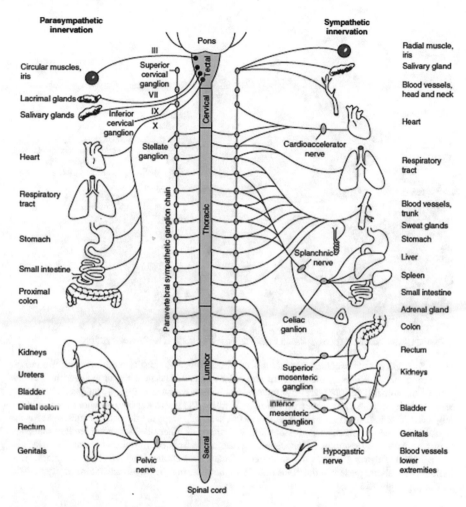

Fig. 6.2 Schematic representation of the autonomic nervous system depicting the functional innervation of the peripheral effector organs and the anatomic origin of the peripheral autonomic nerves from the spinal cord. Although both paravertebral sympathetic ganglia chains are presented, the sympathetic innervation to the peripheral effector organs is shown only on the *right part* of the figure, whereas the parasympathetic innervation of the peripheral effector organs is depicted on the *left*. The *roman numerals* on nerves, originating in the tectal region of the brainstem, refer to the cranial nerves that provide parasympathetic outflow to the effector organs of the head, neck and trunk [from Ruffolo R (1991) Physiology and biochemistry of the peripheral autonomic nervous system. In: Wingard L, Brody T, Larner J et al. (eds) Human pharmacology: molecular to clinical. Mosby Year Book, St Louis, p 77; copyright Elsevier]

the body organs which are the opposite of the parasympathetic system. The presence of cholinergic synapses in this system is important in understanding some of the aspects of toxidromes discussed in Chap. 7.

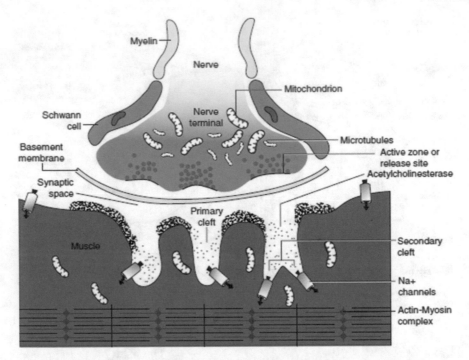

Fig. 6.3 Adult neuromuscular junction with the three cells that constitute the synapse: the motor neuron (i.e. nerve terminal), muscle fibre and Schwann cell. The motor neuron from the ventral horn of the spinal cord innervates the muscle. Each fibre receives only one synapse. The motor nerve loses its myelin to terminate on the muscle fibre. The nerve terminal, covered by Schwann cell, has vesicles clustered about the membrane thickenings, which are the active zones, towards its synaptic side and mitochondria and microtubules towards its other side. A synaptic gutter, made up of primary and many secondary clefts, separates the nerve from the muscle. The muscle surface is corrugated, and dense areas on the shoulders of each fold contain acetylcholine receptors. The sodium channels are present at the clefts and throughout the muscle membrane (from Martyn 2005, p 863; copyright Elsevier)

The special nicotinic synapse that carries voluntary nerve signals to skeletal muscle fibres is known as the skeletal neuromuscular junction (NMJ; Fig. 6.3). This has been the most intensively studied nicotinic receptor whose physiology and pharmacology is known in great detail. Modification of transmission at this junction is part of modern anaesthesia (though curariform muscle relaxants) and a great deal of human experience has been gathered from the everyday use of muscle relaxants by this speciality. The knowledge so gained has been used in the understanding and management of toxic trauma to the NMJ.

6.3.1.3   Essentials of the Processes of Cholinergic Transmission

1. Release of ACh

   When an electrical nerve impulse reaches a nerve terminal, it causes the release of ACh from small storage packages near the membrane of the terminal. The vesicles move up to the membrane and release their contents into the synaptic cleft. Each vesicle contains about 5000 molecules of ACh and each nerve impulse releases about 200 vesicles. The ACh is synthesised within the terminal from choline and acetic acid. The release process is controlled by a number of factors, including a series of proteins known as SNARE proteins (Fig. 6.4), the concentration of calcium in the terminals and also by feedback receptors in the surface of the terminal which are both muscarinic and nicotinic. These ensure that the rate of discharge of the vesicles is sufficient to maintain the chemical transmission which the organs being controlled are working on, for example,

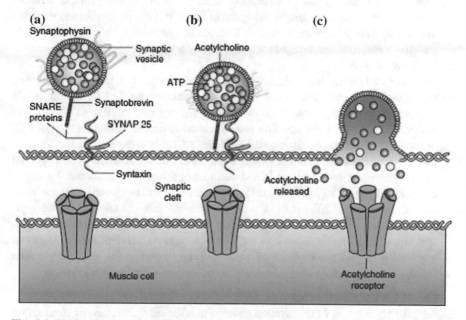

Fig. 6.4 Model for protein-mediated membrane fusion and exocytosis. **a** The release of acetylcholine from the vesicles is mediated by a series of proteins collectively called SNARE proteins. Synaptotagmin is the neuronal Ca^{2+} receptor detecting Ca^{2+} entry. Synaptobrevin (i.e. vesicle-associated membrane protein, VAMP) is a filament-like protein on the vesicle. **b** During depolarisation and calcium entry, synaptobrevin on the vesicle unfolds and forms a ternary complex with syntaxin/SNAP-25. This process is facilitated by phosphorylation of synapsin, also present on the vesicle membrane. **c** Assembly of the ternary complex forces the vesicle in close apposition to the nerve membrane at the active zone with release of its contents, acetylcholine. The fusion is disassembled, and the vesicle is recycled. (From Martyn 2005, p 864; copyright Elsevier)

when a muscle fibre is repeatedly contracting. The amount of ACh released is usually greater than that required to induce an electrical signal in the postsynaptic membrane.

2. Action of ACh at the post-junctional membrane
   When ACh attaches to the receptors on the post-junctional membrane, it causes the channels to open to allow a flow of sodium ions. This induces a depolarisation potential, which generates an action potential and contraction in the muscle fibre it controls. There are many more ACh receptors on the post-junctional membrane than is required to produce an action potential in the muscle fibre it controls. Some of these can be blocked without failure of the junction. In other words, cholinergic synapses have a built-in safety factor which is known in the NMJ as the 'safety margin'. In the case of the neuromuscular junction, the presence of this safety margin is revealed by blocking of receptor sites by muscle relaxants like curare or by alpha-bungarotoxin which is produced by certain snakes. Once the excess ACh receptors which make up the safety margin have been blocked, the released ACh cannot generate a sufficiently strong signal to generate a signal in the postsynaptic membrane to cause the muscle fibre controls to contract. This leads to non-depolarising paralysis of the type induced deliberately in general anaesthesia.

3. Removal of Ach
   After the transmitter has induced a new electrical signal in the post-junctional membrane, it is essential that it be quickly removed so that its action is not prolonged. In nature, this removal is effected by one of the most efficient enzyme mechanisms known. The enzyme used is acetylcholinesterase (AChE) the actions of which are shown in Fig. 6.5a. AChE is contained in the folds of the post-junctional membrane but is synthesised in the liver. It is widespread around the body and is found in red cells from which the levels can be easily analysed. Analysis within synapses is more difficult and not possible in a normal clinical context. AChE exists in parallel with another cholinesterase, butyrylcholinesterase (BuChE) which is equally widespread through the nervous system but whose functions are less well known than AChE. BuChE is important practically in the metabolism of certain drugs, notably the muscle relaxant suxamethonium which is used widely in anaesthesia for rapid intubation.

The AChE-controlled removal of ACh is finely balanced and extremely efficient. The correct functioning of this system ensures that the many millions of cholinergic impulses transmitted throughout the cholinergic nervous system each second can keep flowing. As will be seen later, interrupting this equilibrium leads to toxic trauma over a wide range of organ systems.

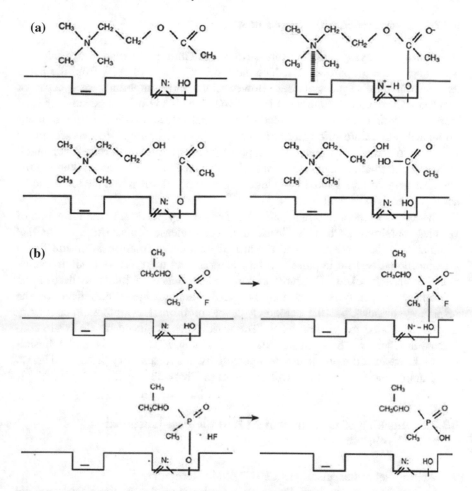

Fig. 6.5 a Normal hydrolysis of acetylcholine by acetylcholinesterase. *A,* acetylcholine molecule and active site of enzyme shown together but not having undergone any interaction. *B,* acetylcholine combined with enzyme to form substrate-enzyme intermediate (short-lived). *C,* ester link in acetylcholine molecule has been broken, and free choline has been formed. *D,* acyl group has become detached from enzyme, leaving choline, acetic acid and enzyme (returned to its original state). **b** Reaction of the nerve agent sarin with acetylcholinesterase blocking the hydrolysis of acetylcholine. Unlike hydrolysis of acetylcholine, reaction sequence is slow because of rate-determining final stage (*3–4*) [from Baker DJ (1993) Anaesthesia in extreme conditions. Part 2. Chemical and biologic warfare. In: Grande CG (ed) Textbook of trauma anaesthesia and critical care. Mosby Year Book, Baltimore, p 1341; copyright Elsevier]

6.3.2   Toxic Disruption of the Cholinergic Nervous System

Toxic agents can interfere with each of the stages of cholinergic transmission given in the previous section involving the release, action at the post-junctional membrane and removal of ACh.

6.3.2.1 Interference with Release of ACh

A number of physiological factors such as calcium levels and drugs such as 4-aminopyridine are known to reduce the level of release of ACh from the nerve terminals in cholinergic synapses. However, the most important toxic cause of reduced ACh release is botulinum toxin (BoTx). This toxin is classically ingested from meat which has been incorrectly tinned and infected with clostridium botulinum and is therefore strictly a cause of severe food poisoning. However, for many years, the toxin has been regarded as a potential agent of toxic warfare given that it is, in experimental animals, the most toxic substance known to man. Although the classical route of intoxication is by ingestion, it is now known that the toxin can be active by the inhalational route.

There are a number of strains of BoTx. They act by preventing the formation of vesicles containing ACh which leads to reduced release. This in turn means that insufficient ACh is released with the arrival of a nerve impulse to ensure that a post-junctional electric impulse will be generated and therefore synaptic transmission becomes blocked. The most striking consequence of this is a descending neuromuscular paralysis which may be life-threatening due to the effects on the respiratory muscles. At the autonomic level, prodromal symptoms such as dry mouth are related to synaptic block. The toxidromes produced by BoTx are considered in Chap. 7. The most important clinical consequence of the pathophysiology of the toxin is the production of a potentially fatal respiratory failure and arrest. More information about BoTx will be found in Chap. 11.

6.3.2.2 Blocking of the Action of ACh at the Post-junctional Membrane

1. Skeletal Neuromuscular Junction (Nicotinic Receptor)
   As noted above, ACh produces an electrical impulse at the post-junctional membrane of the cholinergic synapse which is either transmitted on to another neurone or to smooth or skeletal muscle causing contraction. This occurs by binding of the ACh molecules at special receptor sites which control entry of ions into a channel. At the NMJ, there are two such sites at the entrance of an ion channel in the post-junctional membrane. When ACh combines with these, the channel is opened and there is an ion flow through it leading to depolarisation of the membrane. In the case of NMJ, this causes the associated muscle fibre to contract. The action of the ACh is terminated by AChE. If, however, the ACh receptor sites are blocked, the transmitter cannot attach to them and depolarisation cannot take place. Toxic substances such as curare, alpha-bungarotoxin from krait snakes and black widow spider venom can do this. The overall main clinical effect is the same as for BoTx, namely a paralysis which leads to respiratory failure and arrest. However, the timescale of a post junctional block is shorter than a pre-junctional ACh release block and the

block can be reversed by increasing the concentration of AChE. This type of neuromuscular block is termed a non-depolarising block since depolarisation cannot take place. Controlled blocks of this type with supportive artificial ventilation are a central part of modern balanced anaesthesia. The type of block can be detected clinically using repeated electrical stimulation of the nerve leading to the nerve terminal and produces a characteristic fading response. The electrophysiological characteristics of depolarising and non-depolarising blocks are shown in Fig. 6.6. This can be easily done in an emergency room using a portable nerve stimulator.

2. Cholinergic Blocking at Muscarinic Synapses

   Cholinergic transmission can be blocked at both peripheral and central muscarinic synapses. Blocking at the peripheral synapses occurs with atropine and gives rise to the classic symptoms of atropine poisoning (dilated pupils, tachycardia dry mouth and skin). Central muscarinic synapses can also be blocked by agents such as the incapacitating agent 3-quinuclidinyl benzilate (BZ, see Chap. 3) which gives rise to the central CNS confusion which is a characteristic of the actions of such compounds. As discussed above, blocking of the NMJ nicotinic synapse has profound effects producing neuromuscular paralysis. Equally, blocking muscarinic synapses centrally can also produce important CNS effects. BZ acts as a CNS depressant. Research has shown that individuals receiving an ED_{50} dose of BZ usually develop a full syndrome of delirium and there is very little person-to-person variation. This may be due to an 'all or nothing' action on central cholinergic neural systems.

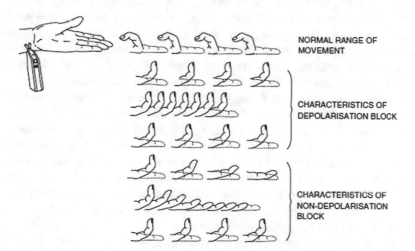

Fig. 6.6 Characteristics of neuromuscular response following repeated nerve stimulation. Depolarisation block, with no fade, is characteristic of failure of neuromuscular transmission in the cholinergic syndrome produced by anticholinesterase compounds such as sarin

As will be seen in Chap. 7, anticholinergic compounds such as atropine play an important role in the treatment of excess ACh following exposure to anticholinesterases. Atropine does not cross the blood–brain barrier and, except in very high doses, does not act centrally. However, a number of synthetic antichoinergic compounds produced as a part of the chemical warfare (CW) development do act centrally producing serious mental incapacitation. The best known of these is BZ. More recently, a possible variant of this, agent 15 has been developed and possibly used. Both agents are considered as potential terrorist threats. Both act in the same way by blocking central muscarinic cholinergic synapses..

6.3.2.3 Interference with ACh Removal

The third way that cholinergic transmission can be disrupted is by blocking the action of AChE, the enzyme responsible for removal of ACh after its release into cholinergic synapses. Toxic substances which do this are termed anticholinesterases. These exist in both the civil setting, as organophosphate or carbamate pesticides or as CW nerve agents which are solely organophosphates. The key to the action of both these classes of compounds lies in their ability to block one or both of two key sites on the structure of the enzyme (Fig. 6.5b). Organophosphates bind to both these sites while carbamates bind more loosely to only one, producing a potentially reversible action. When anticholinesterases are attached to the AChE enzyme, all its action in hydrolysing ACh is lost and so the concentration of ACh builds up in the synapse. The effect of this is to produce a repeated depolarisation at the post-junctional membrane which finally blocks the action of the synapse. At the NMJ, the effect is to produce, again, muscle paralysis but unlike non-depolarising paralysis this time the cause is the repeated depolarisation of the post-junctional membrane leading to an exhaustion of the action of the receptor. This type of neuromuscular block is called depolarisation block and it has different characteristics when tested with repeated electrical stimulation (fade on depolarisation and non-depolarizing blocks). There is no fade on repeated stimulation (Fig. 6.6). Depolarisation block is accompanied by characteristic uncoordinated twitching of the muscle fibres within a motor unit (the group of muscle fibres controlled by one terminal neurone), a phenomenon called fasciculation. Fasciculation is caused by the increased concentration of ACh acting at the nerve terminal. Both fasciculation and depolarisation block can be seen in the anaesthetic room after the administration of the short-acting neuromuscular blocking drug suxamethonium which has depolarizing properties similar to ACh (its structure consists of two ACh molecules joined together).

Increased ACh concentrations in autonomic synapses give rise to a variety of other signs and symptoms which are characteristic of the classic cholinergic toxidrome which is discussed in Chap. 7. The important clinical outcome of AChE inhibition is respiratory failure and arrest. With both carbamate and organophosphate anticholinesterases, this is due to a double action (1) by causing depolarizing paralysis in the respiratory muscles (2) by blocking the initial electrical impulses in the respiratory centres of the brain stem driving the respiratory muscles.

Also in the CNS, increased ACh levels give rise to overactivity of central neurons causing spike discharges and fitting. This is sign of serious anti-cholinesterase poisoning and acts with peripheral NM paralysis to worsen the developing hypoxia.

The ultimate cause of death from all three of these toxic cholinergic mechanisms is type 2 respiratory failure (see below) leading to cellular hypoxia with a failure to produce adenosine triphosphate (ATP), a shift to anaerobic respiration, lactic aci-dosis and cellular death, with the cardiac and CNS systems being the most immediately vulnerable.

6.3.3   Actions of Toxins on the Peripheral Nervous System

The effect of BoTx and the pre-junctional release of ACh has been considered above. In addition, there are a number of neurotoxins acting on sensory and motor nerves. Examples include saxitoxin and blue water algal toxin. These toxins act by blocking the sodium channels in the nerves which lead to a failure of nerve con-duction. In the motor system, this will in turn lead to a failure of NM transmission and paralysis. Paralysis of the respiratory muscles again leads to death from type 2 respiratory failure.

Most neurotoxins cause harm either by ingestion or by envenomation (as in the case of marine organisms and reptiles). However, these toxins have long been considered to be potential agents of CW and were the subject of considerable military research during the Cold War. There are strong indications that some natural toxins can be disseminated by the respiratory route which makes them a potential hazard as an agent that could be used by deliberate release. Further information is presented in Chap. 11.

6.3.4   Non-cholinergic Toxic Trauma of the Central Nervous System

6.3.4.1   Opioids

Opioids are widely used in medicine, particularly in anaesthesia for the control of pain and in producing heavy sedation. They have considerable CNS effects and this has led to their being regarded as potential CW agents in respect of their 'knock-down' capabilities. The actions of fentanyl compounds which may be active by inhalation have been particularly considered. Some of these compounds have an action that is almost instantaneous, causing incapacitation. Opioids act centrally primarily upon the μ receptors. Their actions at the μ receptors can be reversed. The final pathway to death from exposure to opioid agents is again type 2 respiratory failure and death due to cellular hypoxia.

6.3.4.2   CNS Stimulants

In contrast to opioids, drugs such as lysergic acid diethylamide (LSD) which was first investigated in the USA as a potential CW incapacitating agent act directly on specific serotonin and glutamate receptors and also indirectly on other systems such as dopamine, norepinephrine and opioid receptors. There is considerable individual variation in response which led to LSD being discounted as a possible central nervous incapacitating agent in warfare.

6.4   Pathophysiology of Toxic Trauma of the Respiratory System

6.4.1   Mechanisms Leading to Hypoxia

The respiratory system consists of the upper large airways and the lower small airways and alveoli. All levels of this system are vulnerable to toxic trauma from inhalational chemical agents. These may be classified in terms of the anatomical structures affected as shown in Fig. 6.7.

6.4.1.1   Toxic Respiratory Failure

Respiratory failure following exposure to toxic chemical agents has two causes. The first is the failure of oxygen to be able to diffuse across the walls of the alveoli into the pulmonary capillaries and thus into the arteries and cells. The second is the failure of the breathing mechanism to move gas in and out of the lungs leading to a build-up of carbon dioxide in the alveoli. These conditions are known as types 1 and 2 respiratory failure. It should be noted that type 2 respiratory failure has a shorter latency that type 1.

1. Type 1 respiratory failure

Type 1 respiratory failure is characterised by hypoxaemia ($PaO_2 < 80$ mm Hg) with normal or low $PaCO_2$. It can arise from a number of causes, including ventilation–perfusion inequality due to lung parenchymal disease, vascular malformations with right to left shunts, pulmonary embolism and interstitial lung disease, which is the origin after exposure to toxic lung-damaging agents. In type 1 respiratory failure associated with toxic trauma, there is failure of oxygen transmission across the alveolar membrane into the pulmonary capillaries. This is seen in any

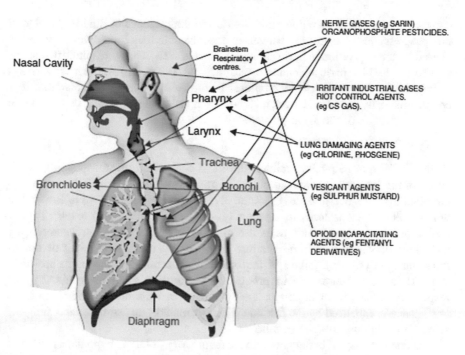

Fig. 6.7   Actions of toxic agents at various levels of the respiratory system

condition where fluid fills the lung sacs (pulmonary oedema) or when the structure of the alveolar membrane is altered. In emergency medical practice, pulmonary oedema is most commonly produced by a cardiac failure and a breakdown of the clearance of fluid from the lungs. This is termed cardiogenic pulmonary oedema. However, inhalation of many toxic agents produces a form of pulmonary oedema which is termed non-cardiogenic or toxic pulmonary oedema (PE, Fig. 6.8). This

Fig. 6.8 Inhalation of many toxic agents produces a form of pulmonary oedema

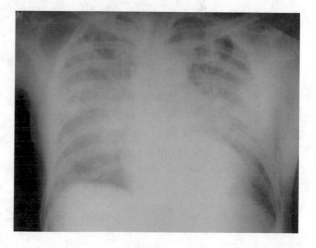

causes type 1 respiratory failure, initially due to the presence of fluid in the alveoli but progressively due to the changes in the alveolar membrane which becomes altered by the deposition of fibrin (fibrosis). This is seen in acute respiratory distress syndrome of which toxic inhalation is one such cause. Type 1 respiratory failure has a longer time course than type 2 failure. In the case of chemical inhalation, it is characteristically produced between 12 and 24 h following exposure, depending on the concentration of the agent inhaled.

2. Type 2 respiratory failure

In this form of respiratory failure (the most common form of asphyxia), ventilation of the lung (the movement of gas in and out of the alveoli) fails, leading to the build-up of carbon dioxide. From the alveolar air equation shown in Box 6.4, it will be seen that this leads to a reduction in the arterial oxygen levels. Type 2 respiratory failure can result from the airways being blocked, for example, by secretions or vomitus or from a failure of breathing itself, as a result of neuro-muscular paralysis or a failure of the breathing control mechanisms in the brain stem. Both these causes can be produced by exposure to toxic agents. Type 2 respiratory failure is an important final pathway in respiratory toxic trauma. Its importance is enhanced by the fact that it can be quickly treated by establishing the airway and starting artificial ventilation.

The end pathway of both types 1 and 2 respiratory failure is hypoxia, a failure of aerobic metabolism in the mitochondria of the body cells.

Box 6.4 The alveolar air equation and type 2 respiratory failure

The relationship between the concentrations of oxygen and carbon dioxide in the alveoli is given by the alveolar air equation. Several modifications of this exist but the simplest expression is as follows:

$$PaO_2 = PiO_2 - PaCO_2/R$$

where PaO_2 and $PaCO_2$ are the partial pressures of oxygen and carbon dioxide in the alveoli, and PiO_2 is the partial pressure of oxygen in the inspired gas. R is the respiratory quotient which has normal value of 0.8.

The level of carbon dioxide is itself proportional to the amount of gas passing in and out of the alveoli (alveolar ventilation) according to the following equation:

$$PeCO_2 = \dot{V}CO_2 \times k,$$

where $\dot{V}CO_2$ is the amount of carbon dioxide released into the alveoli per minute and k is a constant. If carbon dioxide could be removed from the expired gas by absorption onto soda lime (as in the case with certain types of anaesthesia), hypoxia does not occur, provided the minimum oxygen requirement. However, this is not possible in emergency ventilation and so an adequate level of ventilation must be maintained to remove the carbon dioxide produced.

The failure of the normal process of breathing and the flow of gas in and out of the lungs is generally termed type 2 respiratory failure. The failure of ventilation leads to a build-up of carbon dioxide in the alveoli and a reduction in the level of oxygen as indicated by the equation above. In terms of blood gases, type 2 respiratory failure is characterised by a low PaO_2 and a high $PaCO_2$.

In type 2 respiratory failure, the reduction of oxygen partial pressure due to increased carbon dioxide in the alveoli causes less oxygen to be delivered to the erythrocytes and ultimately to the mitochondria. There is thus a failure of the normal cellular respiratory process which generates energy in the form of ATP. Although the cells can move to anaerobic metabolism, this is much less efficient in generating ATP and can only proceed at the cost of producing lactic acid, which is ultimately detrimental to the function of the body cells.

6.4.1.2   Irritant Effects on the Upper Airways

The structures of the upper airway (pharynx, larynx trachea and bronchi) are susceptible to short latency attack by gases which are relatively water soluble. These include substances such as sulphur dioxide, hydrogen chloride and chlorine. The epithelial membranes are affected directly causing rapid inflammation and swelling. Sensory mechanisms are activated which give rise to the classic coughing and choking signs and symptoms.

Due to high water solubility and intolerable mucous membrane irritation, prolonged exposure to these gases is unlikely, unless the patient becomes trapped and/or incapacitated. If, however, there is prolonged exposure or exposure to high concentrations of these highly water-soluble irritant gases, then there can be lower airway injury in addition to upper airway injury.

Chlorine dissolves in water less readily and less quickly than hydrogen chloride. When chlorine dissolves in water, it produces hydrochloric acid and hypochlorous acid which act quickly as a choking irritant on the upper airways. A moderately water-soluble irritant gas, like phosgene, produces effects that are similar to, but intermediate between the effects of the highly water-soluble and the slightly water-soluble irritant gases. In other words, a moderately water-soluble irritant gas produces both upper and lower airway damage. However, the effects are dose-dependent. High concentrations of chlorine produce toxic effects on both the upper and lower respiratory tract and the lung parenchyma.

6.4.1.3 Corrosive Effects

Some of the gases that act initially as irritants have further corrosive effects on the structures of the upper airway. Thus, ammonia dissolves in the water covering mucous membranes to form ammonium hydroxide, a strong base that can produce liquefactive necrosis. Hydrogen chloride dissolves in water covering mucous membranes to form hydrochloric acid, a strong acid that produces coagulative necrosis. Sulphur dioxide has the same effects due to the formation of sulphurous acid. Mustard gas (HD), when inhaled, also produces necrosis of the large airways with blockage due to sloughing of ulcerated necrotic tissue (Fig. 6.9). All these agents will produce type 2 respiratory failure as a result of blockage of the airways.

6.4.1.4 Effects on the Lower Airways and Alveoli

Irritant gases that are slightly water soluble, such as phosgene and nitrogen dioxide, still produce significant irritation to the upper airways which provide a warning of exposure. Phosgene, which followed chlorine as a chemical agent in World War I

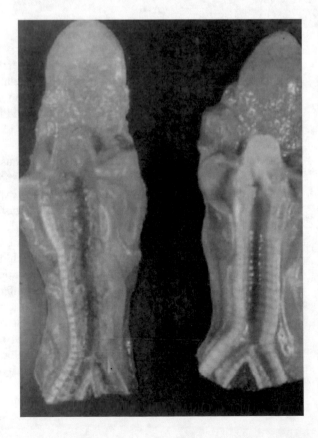

Fig. 6.9 Mustard gas, when inhaled, produces necrosis of the large airways, as shown in the specimen on the *left* of the photograph. (*Source* Medical manual of defence against chemical agents, 6th edition, 1987, HMSO, London)

(see Chap. 2), produced an initial choking reaction similar to that of chlorine. However, the lower solubility of phosgene allows significant amounts to be carried down to the lower airways and alveoli where it causes acute lung injury and toxic PE. These two actions have different latencies, the choking action being almost immediate and incapacitating with PE occurring after 18–24 h and producing a serious and life-threatening action. There is a corrosive local toxic effect on type 1 and type 2 alveolar cells, and on the subjacent capillary endothelial cells, i.e. on the alveolar–capillary membrane, resulting in decreased surfactant production, alveolar collapse and non-cardiogenic pulmonary oedema. This was originally thought to be due to the production of hydrochloric acid from phosgene but experimental studies have not confirmed this hypothesis. In addition to its corrosive action, phosgene acetylates nucleophilic groups such as amino ($-NH_2$), hydroxyl ($-OH$) and sulphydryl ($-SH$) groups in cells of the alveolar–capillary membrane.

The lung-damaging agents provide an interesting example of variation of the Haber coefficient (see Sect. 3.6.3.4), which holds that concentration x time is broadly constant. With gases such as chlorine and phosgene, it is known that the latency of secondary pulmonary oedema is a function of the concentration inhaled. For example, a concentration of 1000 ppm of chlorine is immediately fatal. Contemporary accounts of the April 22, 1915 chlorine attack (see Chap. 2) illustrate the catastrophic and rapidly fatal effects of the inhalation of high concentrations of chlorine. It is likely that the concentrations in the trenches around Ypres were way over 1000 ppm and contemporary accounts confirm that pulmonary oedema was apparently present in some casualties less than an hour following exposure. The classically described period of latency for the development of PE between a short-term, but sublethal, exposure depends on the ambient concentration. For phosgene, it is now recognised that the shorter the period to the development of PE the worse will be the prognosis. This is an important and useful clinical indicator for emergency clinical management and establishment of prognosis.

6.4.2 Mechanisms Underlying the Development of Toxic Pulmonary Oedema and Acute Respiratory Distress Syndrome

The development of acute lung injury (ALI), toxic PE and possible subsequent ARDS is important and potentially life-threatening considerations in pulmonary toxic trauma. There has been a large amount of research in this topic in recent years. Here, we present a summary of the present understanding of the complex pathophysiology of the development of ALI and PE. The management of these conditions and potential protective measure that can be taken in the period immediately after exposure are considered in later chapters.

ALI may be produced by both physical and toxic trauma. In both cases, there is damage to the alveoli increasing respiratory distress and subsequent hypoxia from type 1 respiratory failure. Several aspects of the damage mechanisms causing ALI are clear from the clinical presentation.

1. Simple chest X-ray and computer-assisted tomography scans show initially a heterogeneous distribution of the opacities representing collapsed lung. These can move with a change in posture (Fig. 6.8). Blood gas analysis shows that a major shunt (where blood passes through the lungs without being oxygenated) is evident which usually cannot be corrected by increasing FiO_2. Computed tomography (CT) scans also show areas of lung over-distension which may contribute to increased dead space. The lungs themselves show major changes in mechanics with a decrease in lung compliance (volume/pressure) with ALI from pulmonary causes. There is also an increase in mean total airway resistance.
2. Histopathological studies in ALI show that there are acute and chronic stages. The acute stage is characterised by damage to the blood–gas barrier with extensive damage to the type 1 alveolar epithelial cells. This leads to a leakage of protein-containing fluid into the alveoli together with red blood cells, leucocytes and strands of fibrin. In addition, there is intravascular coagulation in the pulmonary capillaries. In the next (the chronic or proliferative) stage, there is attempted repair of the damage seen in the acute stage. This may lead to the development of acute respiratory distress syndrome. The destroyed type 1 cells are replaced by type 2 cells which do not differentiate into type 1 cells. After a few days, there is fibrosis which ultimately overwhelms the lung tissue and usually leads to death. Clinically, this is shown in CXR and CR scans as the characteristic diffuse opacity of ARDS with severe hypoxia from shunting revealed by blood gas analysis.

6.4.2.1 Cellular Mechanisms of Acute Lung Injury

The complex cellular mechanisms of ALI and ARDS have been extensively studied, but the details are beyond the scope of this text. Readers are referred to specialist reviews listed at the end of the chapter. The essential points are as follows:

Neutrophils play a key role in the development of human ALI and ARDS since they liberate the inflammatory mediators which cause the primary cellular damage. A large number of such mediators have been identified in experimental studies and detected in bronchoalveolar fluid washout studies. These are considered to be four main groups of substances which cause damage. These are shown in Box 6.5.

Box 6.5 Inflammatory mediators in the production of lung damage

1. Cytokines, which include pro-inflammatory compounds such as tumour necrosis factor (TNF) and interleukins (IL). A range of other factors such as IL1, IL8 and also TNF exert feedback on the neutrophils causing further stimulation.
2. Protease enzymes which lead to extensive damage in the lung. Elastase is the most damaging and has broad proteolytic activity on collagen, fibrinogen and other proteins as well as elastin.
3. Reactive oxygen species which can damage the endothelium by lipid peroxidation.
4. Lipid-derived mediators such as prostaglandins, thromboxanes and leukotrienes. These mediators act by amplifying neutrophil activation.

6.5   Asphyxiant Agents

Asphyxiant agents cause hypoxia in the tissues following inhalation without causing damage to the lung structures. They may be divided into the following:

- Active—with a direct toxic action on key systems in the body. These include the following:

  - Carbon monoxide.
  - Hydrogen cyanide.

- Passive—where hypoxia is caused without damage to the lung. These include the following:

  - Carbon dioxide.
  - Oxygen depletion in the inhaled atmosphere.

6.5.1   Active Asphyxiants

6.5.1.1   Carbon Monoxide

Carbon monoxide binds to the oxygen-binding sites in the haemoglobin molecules of erythrocytes. This creates carboxyhaemoglobin and decreases the ability to transport oxygen. When carbon monoxide binds to any one of the four oxygen-binding sites in any haemoglobin molecule, the oxygen molecules bound at the other binding sites in the same haemoglobin molecule are bound more tightly and are less likely to be released to hypoxic tissues. Therefore, carbon monoxide decreases the ability of haemoglobin to both transport and release oxygen.

6.5.1.2   Cyanides and Cyanogenic Compounds

Ionised cyanide has a high affinity for ferric iron (Fe^{3+}) and binds with ferric iron in cytochrome oxidase of the electron transport chain within mitochondria. Free cyanide binds to cytochrome oxidase in mitochondria, interrupting the electron transport chain and decreasing the production of ATP. Anaerobic metabolism, therefore, takes over with the production of lactic acidosis. The actions of cyanide at the mitochondria have a very short latency period.

Normally, there are low levels of cyanide in the body as a result of certain food products and inhalation contamination such as smoking. Small amount of cyanide is normally eliminated using an enzyme, rhodanese found in the liver. Rhodanese catalyses the reaction of cyanide (CN) with thiosulphate to produce thiocyanate (SCN) that is excreted later in the urine. This pathway is one of the means of treating cyanide poisoning as explained in the next chapter.

6.6   Toxic Trauma to the Heart and Vascular System

The heart may be affected by cholinergic effects on the controlling parasympathetic nervous system via the vagus nerve producing bradycardia and asystolic arrest. Equally, the cholinergic system may be responsible for tachycardia and hypertension through the anomalous sympathetic system where cholinergic synapses are intermediaries. This is part of the presenting cholinergic toxidrome (see Chap. 5).

The conducting system of the heart may also be affected by anticholinesterase nerve agents and pesticides producing dysrhythmias and ECG changes.

Many hydrocarbon TIC also have a direct effect on the conducting system of the heart causing dysrhythmias. This is sometimes seen in general anaesthesia, particularly with halogenated hydrocarbon compounds such as halothane.

Finally, the heart has a high metabolic rate and is very susceptible to hypoxia which can be produced from asphyxiating causes given above. Severe hypoxia causes asystolic cardiac arrest secondary to respiratory failure and arrest. This underlines why the early management of respiratory insufficiency following toxic trauma is so important.

Many toxic substances also affect the peripheral vascular system (e.g. ergotamine and several toxins). These effects tend to be chronic, however, and outside the remit of the discussion of toxic trauma as an acute phenomenon.

Short-term trauma to the clotting system is seen with a number of animal toxins, particularly snake venoms.

6.7   Toxic Trauma to the Alimentary System

Toxic actions on the alimentary system may be as a direct action on the structures of the system itself or as a route for absorption of a toxic agent into the body. The alimentary system is perhaps the most familiar form and route of the production of toxic trauma.

6.7.1   Direct Effects

Direct effects include the action of corrosive TIC on the pharynx, oesophagus or stomach. Examples include many household chemicals such as bleach or disinfectants. Many other substances also act as irritants to the gastric mucosa.

6.7.2   Indirect Effects

Indirect toxic trauma arises from the ingestion of contaminated food as in mass food poisoning. Many bacterial toxins act through this route. In deliberate chemical agent release, there is also a risk of ingestion of an aerosolised toxin such as botulinum toxin.

6.8   Toxic Trauma to the Skin and Epithelial Systems

The skin and epithelial membranes are very susceptible to toxic trauma from a number of chemical agents. These range from the familiar corrosive actions of acids and alkalis to the vesication produced by mustard gas (HD) and similar CW agents. Some toxins also cause damage to the skin and epithelial system. Examples include mycotoxins and ricin, both of which have been considered to be CW agents.

6.8.1   Corrosive Chemical Agents

6.8.1.1   Acids

When an acid encounters body tissues, the hydrogen ion dissociates from its accompanying anion (chloride, nitrate, bisulphate, etc.). The hydrogen ion denatures proteins in the cells. This produces a characteristic acid burn where the dermis has suffered coagulative necrosis. This necrosis limits the penetration of the acid deeper into the skin. Heat is generated as the acid is further hydrated (heat of hydration) or as it reacts with proteins (heat of reaction). The released heat causes further thermal damage. Although the injury potential of the acids is frequently associated with their pH or hydrogen ion concentration, other factors are also important. In some cases, the accompanying anion may be more toxic or injurious than the hydrogen ion. For example, hydrofluoric acid is a weak acid relative to hydrochloric acid, but fluoride is the most electronegative element and is extremely toxic reacting with enzymes, cellular membranes, organelles, magnesium and calcium.

6.8.1.2 Bases

When a base encounters body tissue, the hydroxide anion (OH^-) dissociates from its accompanying cation. The hydroxide ion produces a chemical burn termed liquefactive necrosis. Unlike necrosis due to acids, this necrotic tissue is not a coagulum or scab; therefore, this permits deeper penetration of a base into the dermis. Generally, bases are injurious at the site of contact and are not significantly absorbed and distributed throughout the body to produce systemic toxicity. In other words, bases are corrosive, contact toxicants that produce chemical burns at their site of contact because of their local toxic effects.

6.8.2   Vesicant Agents

Vesicant CW agents are compounds that cause blistering and skin necrosis and also affect other epithelial tissues, particularly the bronchial tree. Their action is different from corrosive agents and from thermal injury. Compounds in this class were developed as agents of CW as discussed in Chap. 2.

HD is the most important of the vesicants and has been widely used in warfare in the twentieth century. Although the onset of signs and symptoms is insidious and has considerable latency, the action of the agent is rapid with skin penetration within 3 min. HD is persistent and therefore a danger to medical responders. It has a relatively low mortality but a high morbidity.

6.8.2.1   Actions of Sulphur Mustard

There has been considerable research into the actions of HD. However, this has not so far produced any major advance in the management of HD exposure and no antidote exists. An overall understanding of the actions of HD is, therefore, useful for emergency medical responders but detailed knowledge of the research into the mode of action is not essential to the actions needed to manage casualties.

The target tissues for HD are as follows:

- Eyes.
- Skin.
- Respiratory tract.
- Alimentary tract.
- Bone marrow (an HD burn is considered to be immunosuppressive due to the action on the haemopoietic system).

Stages of toxicity:

1. HD penetrates rapidly into the skin by simple diffusion. There is significant penetration within 3 min and it is aided by humidity and warmth of the skin. Areas (such as the genitalia) with a thin epidermis are particularly vulnerable.
2. HD is converted chemically from bis(2-chloroethyl)chloride (a simple substituted straight chain compound) by cyclisation into episulphonium ions which rapidly attack a wide range of chemical moieties such as thiols, amino and carboxylic groups.
3. These actions target the branches of DNA in the cells causing inhibition of protein synthesis and blocking of mitosis. These actions are both cytotoxic and mutagenic and particularly affect cells that are rapidly dividing (e.g. the base of the epithelium, the haemopoeitic system and the gut).
4. The liberation of proteases leads to the formation of vesicles (see Chap. 8). These vesicles result in an epidermolysis due to cellular necrosis associated with an inflammatory reaction.

6.9   Toxic Trauma to the Blood and Haemopoetic System

The acute effects of toxic agents as chemical asphyxiants in the blood were considered earlier. Most toxic effects on the haemopoietic system such as leucopenia and carcinogenesis are longer term and not strictly within the remit of 'toxic trauma'. However, awareness of the potential longer-term problems emphasises the importance of effective early treatment following exposure to vesicants. Mustard agent, which causes long-term carcinogenesis, is a good example and whose medical management is considered in later chapters.

6.10   Conclusions

The wide range of CW agents and toxic industrial chemicals produces patterns of toxic trauma which can be analysed according to actions on somatic systems. In the case of agents which act upon the central and peripheral nervous systems, there is a good understanding of the pathophysiological mechanisms which has led to a systematic approach to treatment with both life support measures and antidotes. The same is true of chemical asphyxiants such as where the understanding of the mechanisms behind relatively common emergency presentations such as carbon monoxide and cyanide poisoning has produced a range of treatment options. The pathophysiology of lung-damaging agents has been studied intensively in the form of acute lung injury and acute respiratory distress syndrome from both physical and toxic causes. However, while detailed protocols for management have been produced in the case of ARDS, these have largely been derived from ARDS from other causes than toxic exposure. Much of the research has been done on animals and the application of mechanisms so derived to man must be done with caution.

Further Reading

Baskin SJ, Kelly JB, Maliner BI et al (2008) Cyanide poisoning. In: Tuorinsky SD (ed) Medical aspects of chemical warfare. Office of the Surgeon General, United States Army Borden Institute, Walter Reed Army Medical Center, Washington DC, pp 371–410 (Chap. 11)

Eyer PA, Oximes WF (2007) In: Marrs TC, Maynard RL, Sidell FR (eds) Chemical warfare agents; toxicology and treatment, 2nd edn. Wiley, Chichester

Hobbiger F (1976) Pharmacology of anticholinesterase drugs. In: Zaimis (ed) Handbook of experimental pharmacology 42: chapter 4C neuromuscular junction. Springer, Berlin

Hurst CG, Petrali JP, Barillo DJ (2008) Vesicants. In: Tuorinsky SD (ed) Medical aspects of chemical warfare. Office of the Surgeon General, United States Army Borden Institute, Walter Reed Army Medical Center, Washington DC, pp 259–307 (Chap. 8)

Ketchum JS, Salem H (2008) Incapacitating agents. In: Tuorinsky SD (ed) Medical aspects of chemical warfare. Office of the Surgeon General, United States Army Borden Institute, Walter Reed Army Medical Center, Washington DC, pp 411–439 (Chap. 12)

Marrs TC (2001) Organophosphates: history, chemistry, pharmacology. In: Laralliedde L, Feldman S, Henry J, Marrs TC (eds) Organophosphates and health. Imperial College Press, London

Marrs T, Rice P, Vale A (2006) The role of oximes in the treatment of nerve agent poisoning in civilan casualties. Toxicol Rev 25(4):297–323

Marrs TC, Maynard RL, Sidell FR (2007) Chemical warfare agents: toxicology and treatment. Wiley, Chichester

Martyn JAJ (2005) Neuromuscular physiology and pharmacology. In: Miller RD (ed) Anesthesia, 6th edn. Elsevier, Philadelphia, pp 859–879 (Chap. 22)

Maynard R (2007) Phosgene. In: Marrs TC, Maynard RL, Sidell FR (eds) Chemical warfare agents: toxicology and treatment, 2nd edn. Wiley, Chichester, pp 477–494 (Chap. 24)

Sidell FR, Newmark J, McDonough JH (2008) Nerve agents. In: Tuorinsky SD (ed) Medical aspects of chemical warfare. Office of the Surgeon General, United States Army Borden Institute, Walter Reed Army Medical Center, Washington DC, pp 155–242 (Chap. 5)

Tuorinsky SD, Sciuto AM (2008) Toxic inhalational injury and toxic industrial chemicals. In: Tuorinsky SD (ed) Medical aspects of chemical warfare. Office of the Surgeon General, United States Army Borden Institute, Walter Reed Army Medical Center, Washington DC, pp 339–370 (Chap. 10)

Willems JL (1989) Clinical management of mustard gas casualties. Ann Med Milit Belg 3(suppl):1

Chapter 7
The Clinical Presentation of Toxic Trauma: Assessment and Diagnosis

Abstract Detailed information about the released toxic agent causing toxic trauma may not be immediately available to emergency medical physicians. Diagnosis and appropriate early treatment therefore depend on careful history taking and examination. Collections of signs and symptoms, known as toxidromes, have been described and are of use in establishing a diagnosis. However, toxidromes may not always be clear-cut, and there are many individual variations. Signs and symptoms develop with variations in latency. This chapter considers the key practice points in assessing patients who have been exposed to toxic agents and describes the classic toxidromes for chemical warfare agents and toxic industrial chemicals.

7.1 Introduction

Unlike conventional physical trauma, the history and presenting signs and symptoms of patients who have been exposed to chemical agents may not always be clear. In case of accidental exposure in civil settings, there may be a documented history of the incident with appropriate hazardous materials (HAZMAT) measures taken and the agent identified on-site. However, as the Syrian Civil War has shown at the time of writing, the situation in a civil setting in warfare may be completely different with claims and counterclaims that chemical warfare agents have been used but with little, if any, detailed history of the original exposure. Because the use of chemical weapons is banned by an international treaty, any possible use will not be readily admitted by the perpetrator. Equally, the use of toxic agents by terrorists may not be immediately recognised as was the case in the Tokyo subway release of sarin in 1995.

Physical trauma, by contrast, usually has clear signs of what has happened to the patient with penetrating, blunt and thermal trauma. Although other forms (such as blast lung) may be in evolution, by the time a patient is seen by an emergency response team the injuries are usually apparent. This may not be the case with toxic agents where signs and symptoms may be delayed by the inherent latency of the causative agent.

© Springer International Publishing Switzerland 2016
D.J. Baker, *Toxic Trauma*, DOI 10.1007/978-3-319-40916-0_7

Further complications may occur with the presentation of patients who may have both physical and toxic trauma, for example following fires and explosions where there may be burn injury and inhalation of smoke and hot gases.

Due to the relative rarity of release of chemical agents, there may be unfamiliarity among many clinicians with the signs and symptoms of toxic trauma caused by some classes of agents (e.g. lung-damaging agents). However, potential lung injury by smoke and explosions is increasingly familiar. There are also other clinical conditions that will be more familiar to emergency clinicians and provide analogies for toxic trauma. For anyone who is not familiar with toxic agent injury, it is important when examining a patient or particularly a group of patients with the same signs and symptoms presenting at approximately the same time to have a low threshold of suspicion of the presence of toxic trauma caused by deliberate or accidental release of a toxic agent. A lack of suspicion that a toxic agent may be responsible for presenting emergencies has a parallel in the diagnosis of deliberate poisoning. Although self-poisoning is a familiar situation in the emergency department, deliberate homicidal poisoning still remains low in the level of diagnostic awareness.

7.2 Clinical History

7.2.1 Circumstances of the Incident

As with the management of all trauma, taking a good history of the presenting event either from the patient or from eye witnesses is very important. Patients may present with a history of exposure in circumstances that strongly indicate a toxic release. There may be the key signs of a release with unusual smells or the presence of smokes or fumes and the production of multiple casualties. Detection and identification information may be available from the primary emergency responders such as fire services or specialised paramedical response teams where a HAZMAT incident has been declared. This information will be from field analytical equipment and also from sources such as Kemmler plates and the UN identification number as noted in Chap. 3. On-site primary emergency responders, particularly fire service HAZMAT personnel, should also provide as much detail as possible when briefing hospital teams. Box 7.1 summarises questions that should be asked of eye witnesses and casualties.

If a HAZMAT incident has been declared, then the appropriate zones should have been set up and any decontamination required done. However, past incidents show that many victims escape from the cordons and can present directly to hospital emergency departments. In this case, if the patients are contaminated, the potential onward risks to medical personnel should always be borne in mind.

> **Box 7.1 Gathering history of a toxic release**
>
> Patient or eyewitness accounts of the nature of the release:
> Did anyone see or smell anything unusual?
> Was there a fire or explosion?
> Was there an obvious vapour cloud?
> Were there multiple casualties presenting at the same time?
> Were there obvious signs presenting in nearby persons, e.g. convulsions, unconsciousness?
> Were there any identifying features from the source of the toxic release—Kemmler plates, vehicle documentation?

7.2.2   Systemic History

Most established or evolving toxic trauma will be identifiable from signs rather than symptoms recognisable by classic toxidromes considered below. However, low-level exposure may reveal some important prodromal symptoms such as dyspnoea and chest tightness and visual disturbances in case of low-level nerve agent exposure. In addition, there may be other symptoms of upper respiratory irritation. Where possible, a detailed systemic history should be taken, not forgetting a history of any pre-existing respiratory and neurological problems. Patients who have been exposed or think they have been exposed to a toxic release will be very anxious, and constant reassurance will be necessary to gather an accurate clinical picture.

7.3   Physical Examination

Before admission and initial assessment of the patient(s) if there is an advance warning of a toxic release, responding medical teams should bear in mind the possibility of contaminated patients arriving at the hospital. This is very important to prevent further casualties among staff. If the released agent was persistent and there is a possibility that persons presenting at the emergency department may have escaped the HAZMAT incident, security cordon and decontamination procedures outside the department should be put in place. There should be separate lines of admission for contaminated and non-contaminated casualties and this arrangement should be incorporated into hospital major incident planning. Remember that contaminated casualties may require urgent life support and this must be provided by suitably protected medical responders.

7.3.1   Assessing the Patient: Initial Steps

The assessment of a patient with potential toxic trauma should follow the approach taken for the management of physical trauma and should include an initial flash and primary and secondary assessments. In particular, the overall conscious state of the patient and evidence of response together with respiratory status should be assessed immediately.

The flash assessment of the patient should include observation of whether there is evidence of continuing contamination. This may be obvious due to liquid stains and smell. Contaminated clothing should be removed immediately by protected personnel as part of the decontamination process. Removal of contaminated clothing reduces contamination by about 80 % as discussed in Chap. 4.

7.3.1.1   Primary Survey—Key Points

1. The ABCDE system used in advanced trauma life support remains a useful structure for both primary and secondary surveys in cases of toxic trauma, but certain factors in the acronym may have determining effects on the others.
2. Unconsciousness can affect the assessment of disability and the ability to maintain an airway (since the airway and respiratory reflexes may be affected by the unconscious level). The level of unconsciousness in a presenting patient who may have suffered toxic trauma should be assessed immediately after admission, using AVPU and the Glasgow Coma Scale (GCS; see Sect. 7.5.1).
3. Early pre-hospital management should emphasise the assessment of conscious level as a baseline and for the requirement for immediate steps to maintain the airway, even when no equipment is available (e.g. placing the patient in the left lateral position and holding the chin up).

7.4   Triage of Multiple Toxic Casualties

Initial triage of casualties from a toxic agent release was discussed in Chap. 4. It is important to bear in mind that toxic trauma is a developing situation and what presents is not necessarily what will be the situation within a few hours. Frequent re-triage is essential in the management of toxic trauma. At this stage in management, triage should consider what type of toxic agent has been involved in the release as identified from the information about the incident and from presenting toxidromes. Box 7.2 shows triage characteristics of chemical casualties for specific chemical warfare agents.

Box 7.2 Triage features for specific CW agents.

Source Tuorinsky et al. 2008

T1 immediate
Nerve agents
Talking (severe distress with dyspnoea, twitching, and/or nausea and vomiting); moderate-to-severe effects in two or more systems (e.g. respiratory, gastrointestinal, muscular); circulation intact
  Unconscious; circulation intact
  Unconscious, respiratory depression, circulatory failure
  (Note that both convulsions and muscle fasciculation may be seen following exposure to nerve agents. Where there has been skin exposure to liquid agent, localised fasciculations may be seen in the underlying muscle.)
  Cyanide
  Severe distress (unconscious, convulsing, with or without apnoea); circulation intact
  Lung-damaging agents
  Severe respiratory distress with short latency
  Developing pulmonary oedema if presenting after a longer latency period
  Vesicants
  Severe respiratory distress (inhalation of mustard vapour at high temperatures or if adsorbed onto dust)
  Eye injuries (immediate decontamination is required for liquid exposure)

T2 Delayed
Nerve agents
  Recovering from severe exposure after immediate antidote therapy
  Respiratory and circulatory parameters satisfactory
  Cyanide
  Respiratory and circulatory parameters satisfactory 15 min after exposure
  Lung-damaging agents
  Careful observation (ideally for 24 h) following acute exposure with upper respiratory irritation
  Vesicant
  Skin injury >5 % but <50 % (liquid exposure) of body surface area
  Non-liquid eye injuries
  Airway problems starting >6 h after exposure

T3 minimal
Nerve agent
  Casualty ambulant and fully conscious and alert, with no specific signs other than minor chest tightness and miosis
  Lung-damaging agents
  No initial signs of respiratory distress following exposure or developing respiratory problems after 24 h

Vesicant
Skin injury <5 % of body surface area in non-critical areas
Minor conjunctivitis

T4 expectant
Triaging patients as expectant will depend very much on the circumstances of
the release, the number of casualties and the medical care available. Patients
with severe respiratory failure and arrest may fall into this category. Death
will be from secondary cardiac arrest following respiratory arrest. This can be
prevented if early airway and artificial ventilation support is provided.

Key Practice Point At the hospital level, the immediate category should be
identified during the flash survey and life-saving procedures should be introduced
immediately. If the identity of the agent is known, airway and ventilation support
can be supplemented by emergency antidote measures, detailed in the next chapter.
If the identity of the agent is not known and there are clear signs of reduced levels
of consciousness and of respiratory distress, the airway must be secured as a priority, and artificial ventilation from a portable ventilator should be started immediately. Only when key physiological parameters (end-tidal CO_2 and blood oxygen
saturation) have been stabilised should further examination of the patient continue.

7.5   Main Presenting Signs and Symptoms Following
Toxic Trauma

The following notes are intended to emphasise the key features that should be
sought during patient examination following a toxic release and are intended to
supplement the standard medical procedures for examination which will be found in
other texts on the management of the acutely injured.

7.5.1   Nervous System

Primary and secondary assessments must be made:

1. Of the conscious level
   This is done most rapidly by AVPU (is the patient **A**lert, is there a response to
   Vocal commands or **P**ainful stimuli, or **U**nresponsive) followed by a full GCS
   assessment (Box 7.3). This will indicate a central nervous system (CNS)-driven
   need for airway and ventilation management. A GCS of 8 is usually taken to be
   an indicator of the need for definitive airway management (intubation) and
   ventilation, but this should take account of the respiratory state also.

Box 7.3 Assessment of disability using the Glasgow Coma Scaleand AVPU systems

1. Glasgow Coma Scale
   Assessment is made of eye opening, verbal and motor responses.

   Eyes: Open spontaneously—4
   To verbal command—3
   To painful stimulus—2
   No response—1
   Verbal response: Orientated and converses—5
   Disorientated and converses—4
   Inappropriate words—3
   Incomprehensible sounds—2
   No response—1
   Motor response: To verbal command, obeys—6
   To painful stimulus, localises pain—5
   Flexion withdrawal—4
   Abnormal flexion—3 (decorticate rigidity)
   Extension—2 (decerebrate rigidity)
   No response—1
   Total 3–5

2. A rapid assessment of disability in patients can be made using the AVPU assessment

   The patient is:
   Alert and normal
   Responds to **V**ocal commands
   Responds to **P**ainful stimuli
   Unresponsive

2. The presence of convulsions and fasciculations
   These conditions are frequently the subject of confusion. Convulsions are clonic movements of the whole body, most familiar to clinicians as an epileptic fit. Fasciculation is uncoordinated contractions of muscle fibres within muscle groups. A familiar example is seen in general anaesthesia after the administration of the short-acting muscle relaxant succinylcholine.
3. Eyes
   Are the pupils constricted or dilated, and what is the reaction to light? (Note that the eyes should be examined in relatively low-level light conditions.)

4. Is there evidence of excessive lachrymation and acute conjunctivitis (note, if there is circumstantial evidence of the release of a vesicant or a corrosive toxic substance, decontamination of the eyes by irrigation is an immediate priority)?
5. Examination of the peripheral nervous system (PNS) should include the conventional assessment of movements and reflexes to establish whether or not peripheral neuromuscular paralysis is present. Fasciculation of muscle groups as mentioned above is an important sign in nerve agent exposure.

7.5.2   Respiratory System

The effects on the respiratory system (RS) may be a characteristic presentation of toxic trauma and cover a range of seriousness from mild incapacitation to life-threatening cardiorespiratory failure. Because of the problems of the latency of action of many toxic substances, the effects on the RS may be still developing at the time of investigation. Constant re-examination of the systems for signs of deterioration is therefore essential.

As noted in Chap. 4, toxic trauma to the RS and cardiovascular system (CVS) may occur as a direct effect on the lungs and the respiratory tree and also indirectly due to the effects on the brainstem-controlled breathing. Airways may be blocked by direct action (e.g. sulphur mustard) and by pharmacological actions (e.g. nerve agents). Box 7.4 summarises the presenting signs of toxic agents' effects on the airways.

Box 7.4 Ways in which toxic agents can affect the airway

Direct
Oropharynx: sneezing
Nasal rhinorrhoea and excessive salivation
Larynx cough
Laryngeal spasm
Large-airways secretions and blockage
Small-airways bronchospasm, e.g. SO_2
Nerve agents
Vesicants at high ambient temperatures

7.5.2.1 Primary Respiratory Examination

Observation:

1. Is there rhinorrhoea and excessive salivation?
2. Colour of skin and mucous membranes: evidence of cyanosis or cherry red colour?
3. Respiratory rate and form

   Is the respiratory rate less than 8 or greater than 20 per minute?
   Is the respiratory form normal?
   Are there see-saw movements between the thorax and abdomen indicating obstruction or use of accessory muscles?

4. Is there frank bronchospasm, coughing and expectoration accompanied by respiratory distress?

   (If the patient is conscious, ask if there are any respiratory symptoms such as dyspnoea or tightness in the chest? This is often a symptom of low-level nerve agent exposure.)

Auscultation
Auscultation plays an important part in the early assessment of respiratory toxic trauma. It can detect early signs of bronchoconstriction and equally developing signs of pulmonary oedema.
Listen for:
Air entry to the right and left lungs
Wheezing
Rhonchi
Rales (crackles) at the bases of the lungs

The timing of the auscultation after exposure to a toxic agent can provide important indicators about the developing lung pathology. The presence of crackles at the lung bases at 3 h after exposure to a lung-damaging agent such as chlorine has been used as an indicator of the likelihood of developing toxic pulmonary oedema after the latent period. If crackles are present at this time, the likelihood of developing toxic pulmonary oedema is high.

7.5.2.2 Pharmacological Actions of Anticholinergic Agents on the Respiratory System

Direct pharmacological actions of nerve agents on the respiratory system include:

Excess salivation
Secretions
Bronchospasm

Indirect pharmacological actions of nerve agents with effects on the airways include the following:

Convulsions and unconsciousness and loss of airway reflexes
Vomiting, regurgitation and inhalation of stomach contents

7.5.3   Heart and Vascular System

Key Practice Points

1. It is important to perform an immediate check of the blood oxygen saturation using a pulse oximeter (note that cyanide poisoning can interfere with the readings due to the formation of cyanohaemoglobin).
2. There may be bradycardia or tachycardia (both can occur following nerve agent exposure together with hyper- or hypotension).
3. The overall perfusion state should be assessed quickly (pulse >120/min and capillary return >2 s) to determine the possible shock state and the need for infusional support. This is important where there is also associated physical injury.

   The regularity of the pulse, supplemented by ECG evidence should be assessed.

4. Life-threatening dysrhythmia can be produced by a number of toxic agents.

7.5.4   Skin and Mucous Membranes

1. Is there evidence of chemical burning (as opposed to thermal injury)? Look for erythema and evidence of painful areas.
2. Are there developing signs of vesication?
3. If there is evidence of trauma from a vesicant agent, remember that decon-tamination of the eye must be immediate.

Note that there is usually a latent period before the chemical agent affects the skin, and re-examination will be necessary.

7.6   Toxidromes

A toxidrome is a grouping of signs and symptoms which are important in estab-lishing the cause of toxic trauma both individual and collective. A toxidrome can be established only after careful examination of the presenting signs and symptoms as detailed above. Toxidromes can indicate whether the patient has been affected by the deliberate release of any of the six main classes of chemical warfare agents or by one of the five main classes of toxic industrial chemicals

7.6.1 The Nature of Toxidromes

For many years, the identification of specific collections of signs and symptoms following exposure to toxic agents has formed the basis of early medical responses in diagnosis and treatment. This has particularly been the case in the military world for the management of chemical warfare agent exposure. In the civil setting where identification of the released substance may not be immediate, toxidromes have assumed an equal importance and are part of established paramedical pre-hospital response to HAZMAT incidents.

From a medical standpoint, toxidromes may be of considerable value in establishing a working diagnosis following the presentation of toxic trauma and the identity of the released agent where there is presentation of mass casualties. But we should remember that each patient is an individual, and the degree of expression of any standard toxidrome will vary according to the biological distribution that governs toxicological responses. Thus, a toxidrome may be a useful guide and adjunct but should not be regarded as a totally reliable clinical tool. As always, with patients presenting in an emergency, medical assessment of the individual presentation based upon both history and examination should be given priority. Clinicians should not attempt to force the diagnosis in individuals according to the weight of presentations following mass exposure. We should remember that while toxidromes are classical descriptions of primary signs and symptoms following toxic agent exposure, there may be associated secondary signs and symptoms which can confuse a classical toxidrome.

7.6.2 Classical Toxidromes

There is no overall agreement in the literature about the exact toxidromes associated with toxic agents. Approaches vary, depending on the way toxic agents are defined. Thus, some classifications consider 'irritant gas' and 'asphyxiant gas' syndromes which have considerable overlap since both of them cause ultimate toxic trauma through type 2 respiratory failure. In the hazardous materials world, 'corrosive' syndromes have been described while the military focus on a 'vesicant' syndrome to reflect the exposure to substances such as HD.

The following broad toxidromes may be described, based upon the classification of toxic agents given in Chap. 3.

1. Mild and severe cholinergic toxidromes
2. Central nervous incapacitating and knockdown agent toxidromes
3. Syndromes following the blockage of carriage and use of oxygen in the body (chemical asphyxiant toxidromes)
4. Lung-damaging agent and passive asphyxiant toxidromes
5. Irritating agent toxidromes (riot control)
6. Vesicant and corrosive agent toxidromes

These syndromes correspond to exposure to agents which have:

1. Primary effects on the CNS and PNS:

   Anticholinergic agents
   Incapacitating agents
   Knockdown agents

2. Primary effects on external and internal respiration:

   Lung-damaging agents
   Active chemical asphyxiants
   Passive asphyxiants

3. Primary effects on the skin and epithelial membrane:

   Vesicant substances
   Corrosive substances

Examples of toxidromes produced by specific chemical warfare agents are presented in Table 7.1.

7.6.3   Cholinergic Toxidromes

In cholinergic syndromes, the presenting signs and symptoms are related to the build-up of acetylcholine (ACh) in the voluntary and autonomic nervous systems and the characteristic toxidrome has been described for many years. Most cases have been following pesticide exposure or pesticide self-poisoning, but there is also information about accidental and deliberate release of nerve agents.

The following simple acronyms are commonly used to describe the signs and symptoms of organophosphate exposure.
SLUDGE (relating to overstimulation of muscarinic receptors)
*S*alivation and rhinorrhoea
*L*achrymation—with the formation of uncontrollable tears
*U*rination—uncontrolled urinary incontinence
*D*efecation—uncontrolled with diarrhoea
*G*astrointestinal upsets—with abdominal cramps
*E*mesis

Note that this simple acronym does not include the following features of anti-cholinesterase intoxication:

1. Tight chest and dyspnoea (early symptoms)
2. Miosis (an early sign)
3. Bradycardia (from vagal stimulation although tachycardia is more common)
   MTWHF (relating to overstimulation of nicotinic receptors)

Table 7.1 Toxidromes of chemical warfare agents

Agents	Odour	Onset	Symptoms	Signs	Differential diagnosis
Nerve agents	Fruity	Rapid	Weakness, dyspnoea, runny nose, blurred vision, painful eyes	Muscle fasciculations, miosis, wheeze, copious secretions, altered mental state, collapse	OP/carbamate pesticides; cyanide; myasthenia gravis
Blister agents	Mustard/garlic/horseradish	Mustard: hours Lewisite: minutes	Burning/itchy skin, sore throat/painful eyes	Erythema/blisters, haemoptysis/pulmonary oedema	Contact with caustics, sodium hydroxide, and ammonia
Choking agents	Chlorine: characteristic Phosgene: hay/mown grass	Chlorine: rapid onset mild (more severe over hours) Phosgene: 1–24 h	Sore throat/painful eyes; throat/chest tightness; dyspnoea; wheeze	Laryngeal oedema/inflamed throat; pulmonary oedema	Upper airway sepsis
Cyanide	Bitter almonds	Rapid	Painful eyes; dizziness/headache; dyspnoea; collapse	Convulsions; hypotension; rapid, deep respirations; metabolic acidosis and high venous oxygen content	Nerve agents; carbon monoxide; hydrogen sulphide
Ricin	None	18–24 h (ingestion); 8–36 h (inhalation)	Ingestion: diarrhoea/vomiting/abdominal pain Inhalation: cough/tight chest; fever; nausea; weakness	Combined acute pulmonary and gastrointestinal signs	Atypical infections/biological weapons (tularaemia, plague, Q fever), phosgene

*M*ydriasis
*T*achycardia
*W*eakness
*H*ypertension
*F*asciculations and convulsions

7.6.3.1   Interpretation of Cholinergic Toxidromes

Key Practice Points Although the cholinergic toxidromes are a useful guide in diagnosis, there are a number of difficulties inherent in their identification and interpretation. The following points are important:

1. The appearance of individual features of the cholinergic toxidrome is dependent on exposed dose.
2. The order of the signs and symptoms in the SLUDGE acronym does not indicate the severity level of the exposure (fasciculation, precedes depolarising neuro-muscular paralysis and respiratory arrest which is the terminal pathophysio-logical process in fatality).
3. Clinically, nicotinic signs often predominate early in the course of cholinesterase inhibitor poisoning. However, concurrent nicotinic and muscarinic signs and symptoms are often present in both the PNS and CNS. Later in the course of cholinesterase inhibitor poisoning, muscarinic signs and symptoms predominate.
4. Initial signs and symptoms can actually be the result of local effects of an anticholinesterase absorbed through the skin and not from systemic toxicity. Since a systemic dose that produces minimal effects is often only a little less than that capable of causing death, the presence or absence of various signs and symptoms can be misleading, regarding the diagnosis and prognosis.
5. Dermal exposures often produce local effects, including sweating and subjacent muscle fasciculations. Higher doses can cause muscle weakness, fatigue and flaccid paralysis.
6. The major life-threatening signs and symptoms after exposure to large amounts of nerve agents are convulsions, coma and apnoea. Depending on the dose and route, these conditions can develop within 1–30 min after an initially asymp-tomatic period. Convulsions can develop and resolve spontaneously after a short period, or be prolonged and develop into status epilepticus. Apnoea can also be abrupt in onset and must be treated immediately with for example, airway control and positive pressure ventilation together with antidote therapy as described in the next chapter.
7. Generalised muscle fasciculations are common and may continue for some time after other acute signs have decreased.
8. Exposure to small amounts of nerve agents can produce several non-specific CNS effects. Victims of low-dose nerve agent exposures have complained of

forgetfulness, insomnia, irritability, depression, impaired judgment, bad dreams and inability to concentrate. These symptoms can occur in the absence of physical signs. Survivors of large-dose exposures can also develop these symptoms.

7.6.3.2   Cholinergic Effects on the Respiratory System

Key Practice Points

1. Depending on the dose, respiratory symptoms range from the airway obstructional effects of increased secretions and bronchoconstriction with wheezing to the systemic effects of ventilatory muscle paralysis with respiratory failure and arrest.
2. Experimental studies have shown that very low levels of exposure to sarin (Ct 5–Ct 15) produce a sensation of dyspnoea and tightening of the chest without any obvious clinical respiratory failure. At this level of exposure (sufficient to reduce AChE levels in the body by 40 %), there are no other marked symptoms or signs other than a developing miosis.
3. Large exposures to nerve agent vapours can result in severe bronchiolar smooth muscle constriction (bronchospasm), wheezing, copious secretions from bronchial cells (bronchorrhea) and ventilatory failure. At this level, rhinorrhoea becomes a marked sign and the secretions become a major factor in airway blockage.
4. High levels of exposure cause respiratory failure from a combination of flaccid paralysis of the respiratory muscles and a failure of respiratory drive from the brainstem in the CNS.

7.6.3.3   Cholinergic Effects on the Cardiovascular System

Key Practice Points

1. Excessive levels of acetylcholine following anticholinesterase exposure can have a profound effect on cardiac activity. The expected effect on the heart based upon the effects on muscarinic receptors would be increased vagal tone with bradycardia and QT prolongation and atrioventricular heart block up to the third degree.
2. In practice, however, the heart rate can actually increase because of increased nicotinic effects in cholinergic synapses controlling sympathetic release. This leads to tachycardia and hypertension which has been noted as being the most common presentation of nerve agent exposure.

7.6.3.4   Cholinergic Effects on the Skin and Eyes

Key Practice Points

1. Dermal application of liquid nerve agents can produce localised sweating and fasciculations of the underlying muscle. Generalised sweating is a common systemic effect following prolonged or extensive dermal exposure, or after inhalation.
2. Exposure of the eyes to nerve agent vapour exposure usually causes miosis and ocular pain due to spasm of the sphincter muscles of the iris and ciliary body, and dimmed or blurred vision. The eye discomfort is characterised as a sharp or aching ocular pain and can be associated with a mild-to-severe headache. Sometimes, the pain is accompanied by nausea and vomiting. The duration of miosis is variable, ranging from several days to as long as 9 weeks.
3. Note that the presence or absence of miosis does not provide any important prognostic information about the overall response to exposure to an anti-cholinesterase. Experimental studies in humans have shown that there is significant miosis after exposure to sarin at a Ct of only 5. Visual acuity is commonly affected by low-level vapour exposure to nerve agents. The duration of effect, like that of the pupils, can be variable, with normal vision returning within 2–35 days. The assessment of miosis is considered in Box 7.5. Figure 7.1 shows miosis after a low-level exposure to a nerve agent.

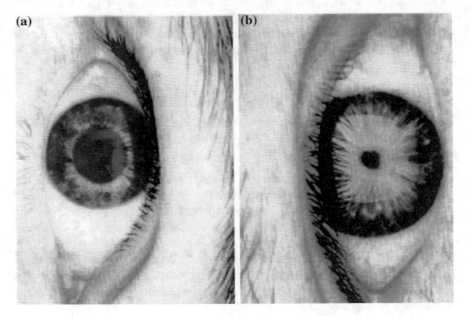

Fig. 7.1 Normal pupil (a) and miosis (b) following nerve agent vapour exposure. (*Source* Medical manual of defence against chemical agents, 6th edition, 1987, HMSO, London)

Box 7.5 The assessment of miosis

Miosis is familiar physiologically under strong light conditions and is a feature of normally reactive pupils. In the assessment of a possible cholinergic syndrome, care should be taken to examine the pupils under low-light conditions.

Miosis occurs at levels of OP exposure which may not give rise to other features of the cholinergic toxidrome other than a tight chest and runny nose.

Experimental studies with the nerve gas sarin have shown miosis to occur at exposure Ct levels between 2 and 5 mg min m^{-3}. At this level, the subjects have reported eye discomfort and difficulty in accommodation.

Experimental studies on the effects of nerve agents (NA) on the eyes have been done by the military to examine the effects of low-level NA exposure on the ability to operate weapons, fly aircraft and think. Performance degradation was recognised to be of great importance after even low-level exposures to anticholinesterases.

This was demonstrated clearly in a civil setting in the emergency room of St. Luke's Hospital, Tokyo, in 1995 after the terrorist subway sarin attack where staff were affected by low-level secondary contamination and had miosis and visual dysfunction which interfered with their ability to work.

4. Equally, lachrymation is not a reliable sign of the degree of early exposure to nerve agent vapour.

7.6.3.5   Cholinergic Effects on the Gastrointestinal System

Key Practice Points

1. Excess acetylcholine increases gastrointestinal motility and secretions. Nausea and vomiting are common findings after inhalation and are usually among the first signs of dermal exposure to a nerve agent.
2. However, diarrhoea may be an infrequent finding. Of the 111 patients who survived the Tokyo subway sarin attack and were categorised as moderately-to-severely affected, only 6 (5.4 %) had diarrhoea. In contrast, nausea occurred in 60.4 % and vomiting in 36.9 % of the patients.

7.6.3.6   Cholinergic Effects on the Genitourinary System

Key Practice Point After both large dermal exposures and the inhalation of significant amounts of vapours, involuntary micturition can occur.

7.6.4   Incapacitating Agent Toxidromes

About 1–2 h following exposure to an incapacitating agent (which blocks central muscarinic cholinergic transmission), the patient presents with atropine-like effects revealed as dilatation of the pupils, dry mouth, increased heart rate, ataxia and drowsiness. After about 6–7 h, there is a confused mental state and aimless behaviour. This phase may persist for several days with bizarre delusions and attempts at self-harm. The syndrome produced is similar to that seen in large overdoses of atropine (belladonna poisoning) although 3-quinuclidinyl benzilate (BZ) is different as a compound in that it easily crosses the blood–brain barrier whereas atropine does not in low doses.

Box 7.6 Incapacitating agent toxidrome

Confusion
Hallucinations
Apprehension
Uncoordinated movements
Blurred vision
Difficulties in urination
Dry mucous membranes
Dry skin

7.6.4.1   Differential Diagnosis of Incapacitating Agent Exposure

Key Practice Points

1. Patients presenting with the signs and symptoms of incapacitating agent exposure may present a problem in differential diagnosis.
2. The possibility that an incapacitating agent has been released must be well in mind when dealing with mass patients presenting with the signs and symptoms shown in Box 7.6.
3. The most important differential diagnosis is that of exposure to opioid-incapacitating (knockdown) agents, since these can have important effects on producing respiratory depression and arrest. The use of an incapacitating agent by Russian special forces to end the siege in the Moscow theatre in 2002 opened a new chapter in the presentation of toxic trauma in the civil setting. Details are presented in Chap. 10. From this incident and from general clinical experience of opioid overdose, a patient will be expected to present with a toxidrome of pinpoint pupils, decreased levels of consciousness and respiratory depression

7.6.5   Chemical Asphyxiant Toxidrome

Following exposure to hydrogen cyanide, the following toxidromes appear with short latency:

Cherry red lips and skin
Nausea
Dizziness and dilated pupils
Severe breathing difficulties with respiratory arrest

Key Practice Points

1. The expression of the classic cyanide toxidrome can be very variable depending on the degree of exposure. For example, there is a wide variation in the perception of the classic almond smell associated with hydrogen cyanide.
2. Following inhalation of a high concentration of hydrogen cyanide, there is irritation of the nose and larynx followed by acute dyspnoea and a sensation of suffocation. This is followed by rapid breathing (Kussmaul breathing) in response to the lactic acidosis created by cyanide.
3. The neurological presentation may be non-specific with anxiety and disorientation occurring at low-level exposures. High-level exposures give rise quickly to generalised convulsions followed by hypotonic coma. The convulsions produced by cyanide may be confused with those caused by nerve agents. In acute cyanide poisoning, the pupils are widely dilated and non-reactive. The dilation is in marked contrast to the miosis of nerve agent exposure.
4. After high-level exposure, the heart rapidly develops multiple extrasystoles, followed by asystolic cardiac arrest occurring within a few seconds of exposure in the most severe cases.
5. In moderate exposures, there is an initial hyperventilation phase followed by reduction in respiratory rate and respiratory arrest. One important feature of early cyanide intoxication is the absence of significant cyanosis, since oxygen carried by the blood is not being used at the cellular level. This gives rise to a cherry red coloration of the skin. If cyanosis is present, this is a very late sign, following respiratory depression or arrest.

7.6.6   Lung-Damaging Agent Toxidrome

Key Practice Points

1. Toxic agents causing upper lung irritation and then pulmonary oedema have strong characteristic smells. Chlorine is the most familiar example.
2. Severe irritation of the eyes, nose and upper respiratory tract gives rise to profound dyspnoea, coughing and a sensation of choking with a short latency

accompanied by nausea and vomiting. These symptoms usually resolve quickly following removal from exposure.

3. Following a variable latent period ranging from 1 to 24 h, there may be signs of developing pulmonary oedema with dyspnoea, coughing and the production of large amounts of foamy sputum (Fig. 7.2).

7.6.7   Irritant Agent (Riot-Control Agent) Toxidrome

In some countries, riot-control agents such as 2-chlorobenzalmalononitrile (CS) gas are frequently used for crowd or riot control. Although the toxicity of these agents is very low, the signs and symptoms of acute exposure are dramatic and may be the cause of an affected person presenting to an emergency medical facility.

Key Practice Points Example: CS gas

1. Irritant gases such as CS gas used for riot control act with a very short latency.
2. There is a characteristic smell followed by irritation in the nose and upper respiratory tract and burning in the eyes with copious lachrymation.
3. There is distressed breathing and a sensation of choking.
4. Except in very rare cases, there is usually no loss of consciousness and respiratory failure.

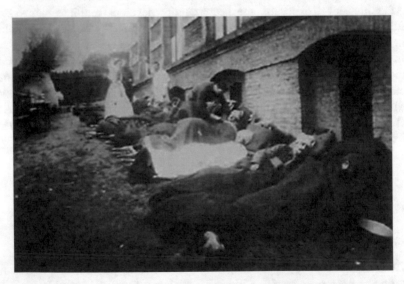

Fig. 7.2 A field hospital during the First World War. Casualties with toxic pulmonary oedema following a gas attack outside a field hospital during the First World War. Little could be done for such cases, apart from providing bed rest during the latent period of possible development of pulmonary oedema following the exposure. (*Source* The National Archive)

7.6.8 Vesicant Agent and Corrosive Substances Toxidromes

7.6.8.1 Vesicant Agent Toxidromes, e.g. HD

1. Signs and symptoms develop with different latencies depending on the ambient temperature. The latency of the appearance of the toxidrome reduces as the ambient temperature increases.
2. Early toxidromes (1–2 h)

   Sneezing
   Itching in the eyes
   Excess tear production
   Eyelid spasm
   Hoarseness of the voice
   Cough (hacking and unproductive in the early stages)
   Shortness of breath

3. Later developments (3 h)

   Reddening of the skin
   Development of blisters
   Breakdown of the vesication with ulceration

   Box 7.7 illustrates these stages of development of the vesicant toxidrome.

Box 7.7 Development of the vesicant agent toxidrome
20–60 min: nausea, retching, vomiting and eye smarting, sometimes no initial symptoms

1 h: first appearance of erythema

2–6 h: nausea, fatigue, headache, painful eye inflammation, lacrimation, blepharospasm, photophobia and rhinorrhoea; face and neck erythema; sore throat, hoarse or total voice loss; tachycardia, tachypnoea

8–12 h: raised erythema (oedema)

13–22 h: inflammation in areas where tight clothing was worn and on inner thighs, genitalia, perineum, buttocks and axillae followed by pendulous blister formation possibly filled with clear, yellow fluid; death within 24 h is rare

42–72 h: maximum blistering or necrosis; coughing appears; mucous and necrotic slough may be expectorated; intense itching of skin; increase in skin pigmentation

7.6.8.2 Corrosive Substances Toxidromes

Exposure to acids or alkalis will usually be identified from a clear history of the event. Toxidromes will present with a short latency and indicate that the patient requires immediate decontamination and treatment. As noted in Chap. 6, acids and alkalis produce different forms of chemical burns. Acid burns form a coagulum and there is evidence of coagulative necrosis. Bases cause continuing saponification of tissues and produce a characteristic 'soapy' presentation.

7.7 Conclusions

Specific toxidromes have been described for several classes of toxic agents and are relevant to both chemical warfare agents and toxic industrial chemicals. Toxidromes may be helpful in establishing a working diagnosis of the class of toxic agent that has been released, particularly when large numbers of casualties present with the same toxidrome at the same time. However, there may be individual variations in presentation, and the features of each presenting toxidrome will depend on the concentration of the exposure. This is particularly true of organophosphate anticholinergic agents. Latency of appearance of the toxidrome may also cause difficulties in interpretation in the case of some agents such as HD.

Toxidromes should be established only after careful history taking and physical examination.

Further Reading

Heptonstall J, Gent N (November 2006) CRBN incidents: clinical management and health protection. Health Protection Agency, London. ISBN: 0901144703. http://www.hpa.org.uk/web/HPAwebFile/HPAweb_C/1194947377166. Accessed 6 June 2013

Tuorinsky SD, Caneva DC, Sidell FR (2008) Triage of chemical casualties. In: Tuorinsky SD (ed) Medical aspects of chemical warfare. Office of the Surgeon General, US Army, Borden Institute, Washington DC, pp 511–526 (Chapter 15)

Urbanetti JS (1997) Toxic inhalational injury. In: Sidell FR, Takafuji ET, Franz DR (eds) Medical aspects of chemical and biological warfare, textbook of military medicine. Borden Institute Walter Reed Army Medical Center, Washington DC, pp 247–270 (Chapter 9)

Chapter 8
The Treatment of Toxic Trauma

Abstract Treatment for toxic trauma may require immediate life-saving resuscitation which should be integrated into continuing antidote and other supportive treatment. For those severely affected by agents with short latency causing respiratory failure or arrest, effective management of the airway and provision of artificial ventilation are key priorities. There are a number of solutions to both, which will depend on the clinical skills of the medical responder, but the most-effective response remains endotracheal intubation and ventilation using a portable volume preset ventilator, capable of overcoming increased airway resistance and decreased lung compliance which are a feature of many forms of toxic trauma. Antidote treatment exists for a number of toxic agents including organophosphates and cyanide compounds. Treatment protocols and continuing investigations are considered. No antidotes exist for lung-damaging and vesicant agents but both proactive and reactive treatment measures are considered, with a view to limiting the possible longer-term consequences from exposure such as toxic pulmonary oedema and acute respiratory distress syndrome.

8.1 Introduction

So far, we have considered the nature of toxic trauma, how exposure can occur and the presentation and diagnosis of those affected. This chapter concerns detailed management of casualties, both in terms of early life support, antidote and supportive therapy, including the specific investigations and treatment required for each class of toxic agent. For a limited number of classes of toxic agent, both military and civil, there are antidotes available. However, in most cases, only general treatment measures are available.

Because of the latency of certain toxic agents, both reactive and proactive approaches to treatment are necessary in toxic trauma, in order to manage immediate life-threatening conditions and also to mitigate developing pathophysiology with a longer latency.

© Springer International Publishing Switzerland 2016
D.J. Baker, *Toxic Trauma*, DOI 10.1007/978-3-319-40916-0_8

8.2   Life-Support Measures

Before any specific treatment starts, there must be a rapid assessment of the
patient's airway, ventilatory and circulatory status. Immediate life-support measures
are required for patients presenting in respiratory failure or arrest and for circulatory
collapse. Patients may also present with both toxic and physical trauma which may
compound the situation. Box 8.1 summarises actions of toxic agents causing respiratory failure.

Box 8.1 Chemical causes of acute respiratory failure

Nerve agents
  Central respiratory drive failure
  Peripheral neuromuscular paralysis (depolarising as part of the cholinergic
syndrome)
  There is type 2 respiratory failure in the case of nerve agent-induced
ventilatory failure with build up of CO_2 and the production of hypoxia
  Other actions of nerve agents on the airways lead to the exacerbation of
respiratory problems:
  Airway blockage from secretions
  Bronchospasm leading to increased airway resistance
Cyanide agents
  Mitochondrial respiratory failure
Lung-damaging agents
  Initial irritant effects and 'choking'
  Possible early type 2 respiratory failure
  Longer latency production of toxic pulmonary oedema and later acute
respiratory distress syndrome with associated type 1 respiratory failure
Vesicant agents
  Direct effects on the large airways with sloughing and airway blockage
  Chemical bronchiolitis and small airway constriction
  Type 2 respiratory failure
  Also possible toxic pulmonary oedema with type 1 respiratory failure if a
dust vector impregnated with mustard agent has been used

8.2.1   Airway Management

In cases triaged as requiring immediate treatment, the airway must be secured
immediately if the patient is unconscious and has signs of airway obstruction.
Simple measures such as tilting the head and lifting the chin and placing the patient
in the left lateral position can be used in pre-hospital care in both the hot and warm

zones (see Chap. 5). The airway may be blocked by heavy secretions and it is essential to use an effective hand-operated aspirator with a wide bore suction tube to remove them.

Key practice points:

1. Suction and immediate airway opening measures.
2. Airway intubation if the Glasgow Coma Scale (GCS) is less than 8. Use of the laryngeal mask airway (LMA) when working in personal protective equipment (PPE).
3. Emergency ventilation management in the case of partial or complete respiratory failure. This must be treated as an immediate emergency. If the airway is not secured ensure that it is open by head tilt, chin lift and ventilate via a pharyngeal mask using a portable gas-powered ventilator (PGPV) or bag-valve device with 100 % oxygen to increase the saturation to >90 %.
4. Continue ventilation using a PGPV with a demand function (to adapt to partial respiratory failure) at 12/min and Vt = 500 mL for a 70 kg person. Ventilation should be at an FiO_2 of 1 initially reducing to 0.5 as soon as adequate oxygenation is demonstrated clinically and by pulse oximetry.

Early toxic respiratory failure will usually be type 2 (low PaO_2 and high $PaCO_2$) and adequate ventilation will reverse this situation quickly. If end tidal CO_2 monitoring is available, this will be a valuable indicator of ventilation effectiveness in this situation.

Note that airway and ventilation must take priority over antidote measures when respiratory failure is present, with the exception of acute cyanide poisoning.

8.2.2   Options for Ventilation in Emergency

The final common pathway for death in toxic trauma is respiratory failure and arrest leading to secondary cardiac arrest and brain death. Therefore, immediate steps must be taken to ensure adequate oxygenation by artificial ventilation.

Emergency artificial ventilation must be provided by a ventilation device linked to an airway device. A number of options exist, the use of which depends on the skills of the responders and experience. Sometimes a combination of airway and ventilation that would not be regarded as offering the best response can produce a significant improvement in oxygenation because it can be applied quickly. Although the endotracheal tube (ETT) offers the best airway protection, if there are significant delays in placing the tube, a worsening of the hypoxia from respiratory failure will result. Figure 8.1 shows possible airway–ventilation combinations schematically.

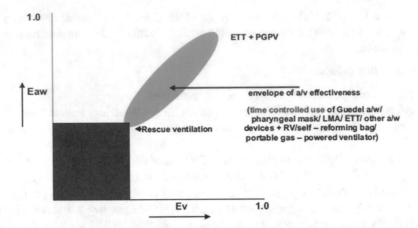

Fig. 8.1 The airway–ventilation (a/v) envelope of effectiveness in emergency response. The *green area* shows effectiveness (Eaw and Ev) of different combinations of airway and ventilation procedures. The most secure and effective is endotracheal intubation and ventilation with a portable ventilator. However, if there is a delay in establishing intubation, this effectiveness is lost and other combinations would have been more effective in overcoming hypoxia. The envelope is a function of availability of equipment, skills in using it and the time taken to commence ventilation. *ETT* endotracheal tube, *LMA laryngeal mask airway, RV rescue ventilation, PGPV portable gas-powered ventilator*. The *red zone* indicates inadequate ventilation due to ineffective application of all airway and ventilation options

8.2.2.1   The Bag-Valve Mask Device

The bag-valve mask (BVM) device (Fig. 8.2) is the most commonly used primary emergency ventilation option around the world. It appears to offer simplicity and rapidity as an option. Ventilation of this type originated in the anaesthetic rooms of operating theatres where it is used to ensure oxygenation on a patient, shortly after induction of general anaesthesia before intubation. In this situation (often where

Fig. 8.2 The bag-valve mask (BVM) device. The bag is fitted with a filter to allow it be used in a chemically contaminated zone

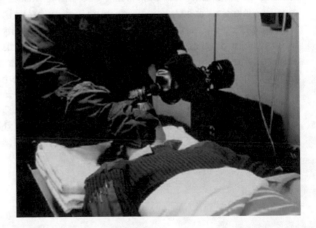

emergency medical and paramedical training takes place), the patient is asleep and has muscle relaxation and an empty stomach. In such circumstances, use of the BVM is usually straightforward and effective. In the conditions of emergency respiratory failure following trauma, both physical and toxic situations are very different with a patient who may still be partially breathing, may have increased airway resistance and decreased compliance and is in danger of vomiting.

In this situation, there are a number of potential dangers in the use of the BVM:

1. There is no adequate Vt, FiO_2 or frequency control. Many devices do not allow the addition of 100 % oxygen to overcome shunting, which will occur in most trauma situations.
2. Therefore, both hyperventilation and hypoventilation are possible. If hypoventilation occurs, the hypoxia will not be corrected.

There is a danger of both barotrauma and volutrauma from hyperventilation. Barotrauma is the busting of lung sacs causing pneumothorax due to too high an inflation pressure. Volutrauma (now recognised as a major contributing factor to the development of ARDS in the ICU) may occur due to the use of too high tidal volumes which cause damage to the alveoli through over-distension.

8.2.2.2 Portable Emergency Ventilators

When ventilating a patient in emergency, there is a need for control in the ventilation to avoid damaging the lung tissue due to hyperventilation and also to avoid insufflation of the stomach when ventilating through an unprotected airway such as a pharyngeal mask. There must therefore be control of the inflation pressure, of tidal and minute volumes and the frequency of ventilation.

These factors can be controlled using portable emergency ventilators which are the devices of choice in emergency ventilation rather than the bag-valve device. A number of ventilators have been produced that are powered by compressed oxygen or by a battery source. Two examples of ventilators specially designed for use in a toxic warm zone are shown in Fig. 8.3.

Desirable Characteristics of Portable Emergency Ventilators In both toxic and physical trauma, portable ventilators should have the following characteristics to ensure that they are capable of overcoming resistance and compliance changes while preventing the possibility of over-ventilation:

1. Time cycled (to ensure a regular frequency of ventilation)
2. Volume preset (to ensure that a correct tidal volume is delivered)
3. Pressure limited (to minimise the risk of barotraumas)
4. Be a flow generator (to ensure that there is sufficient power to ventilate the patient

Pressure-generating and cycled devices are not suitable for ventilation in toxic trauma. Because of their construction, these devices will cycle once a preset pressure has been released. Therefore, if there is airway resistance and reduced lung

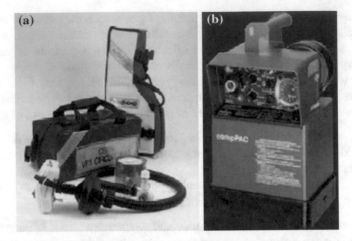

Fig. 8.3 Portable ventilators for use in resuscitation of patients with toxic trauma. **a** the VR1 and **b** the CompPAC field portable ventilator. Both are fitted with a filter to enable ventilation in chemically contaminated environments (photograph courtesy of Pneupac Ventilation, Smiths Medical Ltd, Luton, UK)

compliance, cycling will occur without any significant tidal volume being delivered. High-quality computer-controlled pressure-generating ventilators are more normally used in hospital settings where they can be adapted carefully to the patients' lung conditions. These have a role in the longer-term intensive care of some cases of respiratory toxic trauma.

8.2.3   Circulation

As noted in Chap. 6, toxic trauma can affect the heart and major vessels in a number of ways. A hypodynamic circulation with low blood pressure and poor central perfusion is potentially life-threatening as it is with hypovolaemic shock in physical trauma. Many chemical warfare (CW)/toxic industrial chemicals (TIC) agents give rise to potentially life-threatening cardiac dysrhythmias, for example, organophosphate (OP) agents and hydrocarbons. Profound hypoxia may cause secondary asystolic cardiac arrest which is the end stage of most toxic trauma.

Key practice points:

1. Establish vascular access. Intravenous access is difficult when wearing PPE and intraosseous access offers a better alternative which has been adopted by a number of emergency services.
2. Pharmacological support should be provided following advanced cardiac life-support guidelines.
3. Constant monitoring of pulse, electrocardiography (ECG) and blood pressure is essential.

8.3 Specific Treatment Measures for Toxic Trauma

8.3.1 Management of Nerve Agent Exposure

Key practice points:

1. Nerve agents have a short latency and can rapidly produce life-threatening effects. The immediate assessment of a nerve agent victim should focus on the patient's clinical condition and the route of exposure as noted in Chap. 7. Vapour exposure usually causes immediate symptoms. Symptom onset can be significantly delayed after dermal exposure.
2. Resuscitation with airway clearance and artificial ventilation must begin immediately following a significant inhalational exposure. Life-threatening symptoms can begin less than 5 min after exposure and death can occur within 5 min after the onset of seizures and respiratory arrest.
3. Atropine and pralidoxime are essential antidotes for the resuscitation and treatment of victims of nerve agent poisoning. Control of convulsions, if there is a significant central nervous system (CNS) involvement, must be achieved quickly with benzodiazepines.

Box 8.2 summarises the approach towards the emergency clinical management of nerve agent poisoning.

> **Box 8.2 Emergency management of nerve agent exposure**
>
> Airway
>
> 1. The airway is vulnerable to blockage by secretions, vomitus and bronchospasm. The first step in controlling the airway is by simple measures (head tilt–chin lift). Since there is an excessive production of secretions from the muscarinic effects, effective suctioning of the airway is essential in the early stages of management. The sucker used should preferably be hand operated and of the pistol grip type and with a wide bore suction tube that can cope with thick secretions and vomitus. Narrow bore, gas-powered suckers are unsuitable. Atropine will reduce the secretions in time but suctioning is vital in the early stages of management.
> 2. Establish a definitive airway if ventilation is necessary by (1) LMA or (2) intubation. This will depend on the available skill level. Supraglottic devices are more easily inserted if the operator is wearing a personal protective equipment including gloves. While not providing as secure an airway as an ETT, the speed of insertion and access to the main airway is a considerable advantage. The use of an intubating LMA facilitates the insertion of an ETT in difficult cases. Atropine should be given only after adequate oxygenation has been established in case of respiratory failure. Serious dysrhythmias can be associated with hypoxia.

Breathing

Assess the breathing rate, form and depth. Look for signs of peripheral and central cyanosis. If the patient is still breathing, free-flow oxygen may be used to ensure oxygenation. Patients with inadequate spontaneous ventilation should be ventilated initially with a BVM and 100 % oxygen followed by ventilation using a volume preset portable ventilator. Care must be taken not to over inflate the lungs when a BVM is used.

Cardiovascular

1. Following initial assessment of pulse and blood pressure, the patient should be placed on a cardiac monitor and monitored for dysrhythmias. If these occur, they should be treated according to advanced cardiac life-support (ACLS) guidelines.
2. Haemodynamically, significant bradycardia (i.e. bradycardia occurring concurrently with hypotension) should be treated with atropine by titration. Most patients can be managed with 4–6 mg of atropine.
3. Severe hypoxia should be corrected before using atropine to avoid production of life-threatening dysrhythmias.

Disability (Nervous System)

The patient's level of consciousness should be assessed continually using the alert, voice, pain, unresponsiveness (AVPU) or GCS systems. If seizures develop, despite adequate oxygenation and blood glucose, then treat the seizures immediately with intravenous (IV) diazepam or lorazepam.

Exposure

After skin contact with nerve agents, in their liquid states, ensure that the patient has been undressed and adequately decontaminated in the field with copious amounts of water and a mild liquid detergent, or a dilute 0.5 % sodium hypochlorite (bleach) solution, for at least 15 min.

8.3.1.1   Antidote Administration

Atropine Atropine is indicated in most cases of organophosphate CW agent exposure and for organophosphate and carbamate pesticide poisoning. There is a large body of human data available in the latter case. Atropine is derived from the plant Atropa belladonna (or deadly nightshade). It was used by ladies of fashion in the eighteenth century to dilate their pupils and thus increase their allure. Its main use in non-toxic practice in modern medicine is in anaesthesia to block the anticholinergic effects of neostigmine, a carbamate anticholinesterase used to reverse the actions of non-depolarising muscle relaxants.

The following points are important in the use of atropine in anticholinesterase poisoning:

1. Atropine is a symptomatic antidote for the muscarinic signs and symptoms of anticholinesterase poisonings. Atropine is a parasympatholytic and works only at the muscarinic receptors. It does not counteract the effects of excess acetylcholine at nicotinic receptors. Therefore, atropine cannot counteract fasciculations, weakness, flaccid paralysis or respiratory arrest that is due to neuromuscular blockade at nicotinic receptors.
2. Atropine does not regenerate acetylcholinesterase which is bound to an anticholinesterase.
3. The total doses of atropine for nerve agent poisoning are often much smaller than those needed to treat organophosphate insecticide poisoning. This is because organophosphate insecticides are more slowly metabolised and more lipid soluble. Consequently, they are cleared much more slowly from the body; therefore, the cumulative dose of atropine can reach much higher totals as revealed by management of OP pesticide poisoning in India and other countries.

Atropine indications and dosage:

1. Atropine should be reserved to treat moderate-to-severe signs and symptoms of OP poisoning.
2. Mild exposures to anticholinesterases resulting only in miosis do not require atropine. Atropine does not necessarily reverse miosis, and it can cause other problems such as heat stress.
3. Miosis and ciliary spasm with severe eye pain can be treated with topical homatropine ophthalmic drops, if necessary.
4. Rhinorrhoea generally does not merit atropine administration, unless it is severe and interferes with the patient management.
5. Moderate airway discomfort from bronchospasm and increased secretions should be treated with atropine, 1–2 mg IV or intramuscular (IM), and repeated, as needed, every 5–10 min, until breathing is easier.
6. In severe cases of nerve agent poisoning, atropine should be given as an initial dose of 6 mg IV or IM and then 2 mg IV or IM, every 5–10 min, until breathing has improved and secretions have dried.
7. The indications to treat children with atropine are the same as those in adults. Paediatric doses of atropine must be adjusted for weight and age as follows:

Infant (<2 years old): 0.5 mg maximum single dose, repeated as clinically indicated.

Child (2–10 years old): 1.0 mg maximum single dose, repeated as clinically indicated.

Adolescent: 2.0 mg maximum single dose, repeated as clinically indicated.

Atropine is typically dispensed in 2 mg ampoules but larger doses are available for mass casualty use in some countries. In the military setting, atropine is available to combatants in the form of an autojector. Autojectors are automatic IM injection

Fig. 8.4 An early NATO autoinjector device containing atropine and pralidoxime. The cap contained 5 mg diazepam which was taken orally to treat convulsions. Later models contained lysine diazepam in solution with the other components

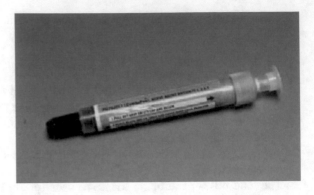

devices that were developed by the military to allow rapid self-administration of antidotes on the battlefield. Typically, an autojector contains atropine, pralidoxime and a diazepine (Fig. 8.4).

Side effects of atropine administration:

1. If there is an excess of acetylcholine following anticholinesterase exposure, the administration of atropine should produce no ill effects. However, excessive amounts of atropine, either from giving too much to a symptomatic patient or from giving atropine to an unexposed person, can produce anticholinergic effects such as dry mouth, blurred vision, dilated pupils, urinary retention, tachycardia and inability to sweat. These side effects are generally considered minor, but they can last for 24–48 h.
2. Significant caution should be exercised when hypoxia is present in cases of severe nerve agent poisoning since atropine can cause serious dysrhythmias in this situation. As noted above, the hypoxia should be corrected by free-flow oxygen or artificial ventilation before giving atropine.
3. However, atropine should not be withheld from a victim of severe nerve poisoning because of a concern about precipitating a life-threatening dysrhythmia, especially if the victim is an apparently healthy young person with an otherwise healthy heart.

Because of its use in OP pesticide poisoning, much has been published about the doses of atropine required, which in some cases can be very high in order to contain a persistent bradycardia. The reader is referred to specialised texts listed at the end of the chapter for more details.

Oximes Oximes are compounds capable of reactivating, in some cases the complex formed by the OP compounds and acetylcholinesterase. Chemically, oximes are mono or bispyridinium compounds which can bind to the OP–AChE complex and cause the nerve agent molecule to separate from the enzyme. Importantly, oximes can reverse the actions of OP at both muscarinic and nicotinic receptors. Thus, unlike atropine, they act at the neuromuscular junction and can thus reduce the degree of paralysis. They have been shown to be effective in the management of OP pesticide poisoning. However, their effectiveness against nerve agents is dependent on the compound involved and on the length of time after the attack before they are given. This is because chemical changes take place in the nerve agent–enzyme complex known as 'ageing'. Ageing occurs very rapidly in man following exposure to the nerve agent soman (GD) but less so in the other nerve agents, for example, sarin.

Although a number of oximes have been synthesised and tested, only two, pralidoxime and obidoxime, are widely used in civilian practice.

Pralidoxime (2-PAM) Pralidoxime is a commonly used oxime and is recommended for all cases of moderate-to-severe nerve agent poisoning. The optimal dosage is dependent on the nerve agent, time since exposure and the cholinesterase activity of the victim. There has been considerable experience with pralidoxime and other oximes over many years in the treatment of OP pesticide poisoning.

Details of the dosage of pralidoxime are given in Box 8.3.

Box 8.3 Use of pralidoxime

The recommended dose of pralidoxime for nerve agent exposure is variable, depending on the route of exposure and the severity of the poisoning.

Oxime therapy should be given simultaneously with atropine. Slow IV injection of pralidoxime is recommended to prevent laryngospasm, muscle rigidity and hypertension. Pralidoxime 15–30 mg/kg IV/IM is given over 20 min for adults and children. In practice, this means 1–2 g dosage (in 250 mL of normal saline), over 5–10 min, for a 70 kg person. This dose may be repeated after 4 h (or 1 h if paralysis is worsening). The target therapeutic blood concentration should be 4 µg/mL. Oxime treatment in hospital should continue for as long as atropine is required.

2-PAM is rapidly excreted unchanged in the urine, with 80–90 % of an IM or IV dose excreted within 3 h.

Pralidoxime complications In a case of true cholinergic crisis, no side effects are expected from the administering of 2-PAM. When pralidoxime is given to healthy adults without nerve agent toxicity, it can cause brief side effects such as dizziness and blurred vision. Hypertension is the side effect of greatest concern. Hypertension can occur with normal doses and recommended infusion rates. At doses of 45 mg/kg, systolic pressures can increase by >90 mm Hg and diastolic pressures can increase by 30 mm Hg. These elevations can persist for several hours. Increasing the infusion time to 30–40 min can minimise this potential side effect.

Obidoxime Obidoxime (Toxogonin) is widely used in some countries for OP exposure but there has been considerable debate about whether it is superior to pralidoxime.

Obidoxime and pralidoxime have been shown in animal studies to be effective against sarin and VX poisoning in different species but both are ineffective against cyclosarin. Obidoxime has been shown to be superior to pralidoxime and HI-6 (a recently developed oxime used in the military setting) for tabun poisoning.

Obidoxime should be given by slow IV infusion of 250 mg.

Side effects of obidoxime In human studies, obidoxime 250 mg IM has been reported to be associated with a hot, tight feeling in the orofacial region associated with numbness. 'Cold sensations' have also been reported in the rhino-pharyngeal region—a sensation rather like that of inhaling menthol. Some changes in systolic and diastolic blood pressure have been reported, together with tachycardia.

Managing nerve agent-induced convulsions Patients exhibiting convulsions following nerve agent exposure should be treated as quickly as possible using a benzodiazepine compound. Diazepam has been used for many years and included in military autojectors in a form compounded with lysine to improve solubility. Central convulsions can worsen cerebral hypoxia which has been precipitated by respiratory failure. The use of benzodiazepines must therefore be associated with respiratory support.

8.3.1.2 The Importance of Respiratory Support in the Management of Severe Anticholinesterase Exposure

Clinically, experience of the management of nerve agent exposure is limited to that gained during the Iran–Iraq war and from the 1995 Tokyo sarin incident (see Chap. 10). However, there is a great deal of experience, both emergency and in the ICU, from the management of OP pesticide poisoning which also produces a cholinergic depolarising paralysis with usually a different time course from nerve agents. In pesticide poisoning, there is established clinical evidence of returning spontaneous ventilation after a few hours in conjunction with anticholinergic and oxime therapy. Patients who were completely paralysed during a cholinergic syndrome will have gradually returning respiratory drive and will fight the ventilator with their own breathing efforts. As noted earlier, modern portable ventilators have a demand valve system to overcome this problem, allowing the ventilator to adapt to the patient's own respiratory efforts. When normal breathing returns, the operation of the ventilator is suppressed and 100 % oxygen is delivered in synchrony with the patient breaths.

Box 8.4 summarises the management of nerve agent exposures in terms of the clinical effects produced. It is important that the treatment given should match the severity of the signs and symptoms displayed.

> **Box 8.4 Management of nerve agent exposures in terms of the clinical effects produced**
>
> **Mild Effects:**
>
> 1. Inhalational Exposure:
>
> If the exposure was to a volatilised agent and the symptoms are minor, then observe for 2–4 h. For patients with chest tightness or upper airway

secretions that are not resolving, give atropine 2.0 mg IM or IV and 600 mg 2-PAM or 1 g IV over 5–10 min.

2. Dermal Exposure:

If there is local sweating or muscle fasciculations at the exposure site within 2 h of a dermal exposure, then give atropine 2.0 mg IM or IV and 2-PAM 600 mg IM or 1 g IV over 5–10 min. Observe for at least 18 h.

Moderate Effects:

1. Inhalational Exposure:

If there is a significant respiratory distress, muscle weakness, muscle fasciculations or gastrointestinal symptoms, then give an initial dose of atropine, 4.0 mg IM or IV and 1200 mg.

2. Dermal Exposure:

If moderate symptoms such as vomiting and diarrhoea occur within several hours after percutaneous exposure, then give atropine 4.0 mg IM or IV and 1200 mg of 2-PAM IM or 1–2 g IV over 5–10 min. Repeat 2.0 mg doses of atropine may be given, as needed, as well as 2-PAM up to a maximum of 3 g via bolus dosing. Onset of gastrointestinal symptoms more than 6 h after exposure can be treated adequately with 2.0 mg atropine IM or IV and 600 mg of 2-PAM IM or 1 g IV over 5–10 min. Observe for at least 18 h.

Severe Effects:

Inhalation or Dermal Exposure:

Establishing an airway with adequate ventilation and oxygenation is the first priority.

Give atropine 6.0 mg IM or IV. Give additional atropine 2.0 mg, every 3–5 min, until secretions have dried and possible bradycardia is controlled. A total of 15–20 mg might be required over the first 3 h. Give 1800 mg of 2-PAM IM or 2 g IV over 5–10 min, repeated up to every hour, if needed, to a total of 3 g via bolus dosing. Diazepam or lorazepam should be used to control patients with epileptiform seizures.

8.3.2 Management of Incapacitating Agent Exposure

8.3.2.1 Centrally Acting Anticholinergic Agents

Anticholinergic incapacitating agents such as 3-quinuclidinyl benzilate (BZ) cause hyperactivity and confusion, which must be controlled as quickly as possible to prevent the patient from harming himself. In severe cases, airway and ventilation management may be necessary.

Physostigmine (a naturally occurring carbamate anticholinesterase compound extracted from the Calabar bean) may be used as an antidote to the effects of BZ. It should be administered intravenously with care in severely affected patients in doses of 2–4 mg given at hourly intervals.

8.3.2.2   Management of Knockdown Agent Exposure

Knockdown agents are a special form of incapacitating agent which rapidly produces an anaesthetic-like state following inhalation. There is one substantiated case of such agents being used in the civil setting, namely the 2002 Moscow Theatre incident, where the Russian special forces claimed they used a powerful opiate compound (a fentanyl). Fatalities occurred from respiratory failure and arrest (see Chap. 10).

In the management of an opiate knockdown agent exposure, early airway and ventilation assessment is essential and intermittent positive pressure ventilation with 100 % oxygen should start as soon as possible if there is a respiratory failure. An antidote to the respiratory depression caused by opiates is naloxone which is used both in anaesthetic and clinical toxicological practice. This is given in doses of 0.4 mg IV repeated until there is a reversal of the respiratory depression. It should be noted that in cases of mixed injury where opioids may have been given for pain relief, the analgesic effect will also be reversed.

Artificial ventilation must be continued while naloxone is being administered until the patient has a sufficient respiratory effort. This can be detected clinically and by using a portable ventilator with a demand function set to continuous mandatory ventilation (CMV) demand. The Moscow theatre incident (see Chap. 10) showed the lethal effects of opioids on respiration and the dangers of relying on antidote therapy alone.

8.3.3   Management of Cyanide Agent Exposure

8.3.3.1   General Points of Management

1. Cyanide compounds are chemical asphyxiants that act with a very short latency. There must therefore be a rapid initial assessment and resuscitation for nerve agents. Ensure adequate ventilation with 100 % oxygen for symptomatic patients. Adequate ventilation with 100 % oxygen helps diminish the absorption of inhaled hydrogen cyanide gas or gaseous cyanogenic compounds, such as cyanogen or cyanogen chloride.

2. Note that in the clinical assessment of hypoxia, skin colour assessment complicated by the presence of cyanohaemoglobin produces a cherry red colouration to the skin.

Box 8.5 summarises the essential stages in the management of cyanide exposure

---

Box 8.5 Stages in the treatment of cyanide exposure

- Chemical antidotes are usually not required if the patient is breathing normally and is fully conscious 5 min after removal from the exposure site. Recovery should be spontaneous with oxygen therapy and reassurance.
- If there is a suspicion that the patient has been exposed to cyanide in liquid form, ensure that either they have been decontaminated or that the responding medical team is equipped with personal protective equipment.
- Establish and maintain airway; give high flow oxygen by non-rebreathing mask; intubate or insert LMA and ventilate.
- If there is a liquid contamination of patient or clothing, quickly remove clothing if not already done (double-bag, seal, label and store securely); decontaminate using shower or wash–wipe–rinse with liquid soap and water; remove contact lenses if present and possible without eye damage and gently irrigate eyes with lukewarm water or 0.9 % NaCl solution; check triage tags for details of pre-hospital treatment.
- Establish IV access with large-bore cannula; monitor ECG; correct acidosis with sodium bicarbonate IV.
- If a cyanide compound has been ingested, do not induce vomiting. If less than 1 h since ingestion activated, charcoal slurry or gastric lavage may be used.
- In hospital practice, take 5–10 mL blood into lithium heparin or plastic tube for blood cyanide level before giving chemical antidotes.
- If respiratory depression and/or impaired consciousness is present (Glasgow Coma Scale less than 8 or U in AVPU rating) and antidotes are not already given, give them in association with artificial ventilation.

8.3.3.2   Antidotes

A primary goal in management is to remove cyanide from cytochrome oxidase so aerobic metabolism can resume. Since cyanide has a higher affinity for ferric iron, sodium nitrite is administered to oxidise haemoglobin (Fe^{2+}) to methaemoglobin (Fe^{3+}).

Fifty per cent of all iron in humans is present as ferrous iron (Fe^{2+}) in haemoglobin. Only 0.5 % of all iron in humans is present as ferric iron (Fe^{3+}) in cytochrome oxidase, an enzyme in the mitochondria. Therefore, the body has a large reservoir of ferrous iron in haemoglobin that can be changed to ferric iron-producing methaemoglobin that binds cyanide and releases cyanide from cytochrome oxidase.

Another primary goal is to convert cyanide to the much less toxic thiocyanate. Sodium thiosulphate accelerates this detoxification of cyanide to thiocyanate.

The treatment schedule is as follows:

1. Sodium nitrite with sodium thiosulphate:

   – Adult: 10 mL of 3 % sodium nitrite IV over 5–20 min; followed by 25 mL of 50 % sodium thiosulphate IV over 10 min
   – Child: 4–10 mg/kg body wt max. 300 mg (0.13–0.33 mL/kg, max. 10 mL) 3 % sodium nitrite IV; then sodium thiosulphate
   – 400 mg/kg body wt max. 12.5 g (=0.8 mL/kg max. 25 mL of 50 % solution) over 10 min

2. Chelating agents

A further approach in antidote management is to use chelating compounds which actively bind the cyanide and are then excreted in the urine. The main agent in use is Kelocyanar (dicobalt edetate). Careful consideration should be given before this antidote is used. If there has been no exposure to cyanide, there may be serious adverse effects include vomiting; facial, laryngeal and pulmonary oedema; anaphylaxis, severe hypotension.

The treatment schedule is as follows:

• Adult: Dicobalt edetate 300 mg (1 ampoule = 20 mL of 15 mg/mL) IV over 1 min followed by 50 mL glucose 50 % (500 mg/L) IV
• Child: Dicobalt edetate 0.5 mL/kg of 15 mg/mL solution (=7.5 mg/kg) IV over 1 min, then 2.5 mL glucose 50 % IV for each mL of dicobalt edetate

If no response, repeat once and re-evaluate the diagnosis.

Hydroxocobalamin
This antidote is used widely in some countries and has been shown to be effective in cyanide exposure from products of combustion.

The treatment schedule is as follows:

Adults: 5–10 g reconstituted in 100 mL normal saline
Child: 70 mg/kg
NB: Hydroxocobalamin causes a bright red coloration in the blood.

A summary of antidote treatments for cyanide poisoning is shown in Table 8.1.

Table 8.1 Management of exposure to hydrogen cyanide

Therapy	Mechanism	Route	Dose	Concurrent drugs	Admin time	Potential antidote toxicity
Oxygen	Increased arterial O_2 content, potentiates activity of other antidotes	Inhalation via mask or endotracheal tube (ETT)	High flow via mask or 100 % via ETT Intermittent positive pressure ventilation if respiratory failure and arrest		No more than 24 h	Unlikely—possible in patients with chronic obstructive pulmonary disease (COPD)
Sodium nitrite	Methaemoglobin formation	Intravenous injection	Adult: 300 mg (10 mL of 30 mg/mL 3 %) Child: 0.13–0.33 mL/kg of 30 mg/mL (3 %) solution (i.e 4 mg to 10 mg/kg body weight)	Adults: sodium thiosulphate 25 mL of 500 mg/mL, (50 %) solution and oxygen Child: sodium thiosulphate 1.65 mL/kg body weight of 250 mg/mL (25 %) solution (approx. 400 mg/kg body weight) and oxygen	No less than 5 min and up to 20 min	Methaemoglobinaemia, vasodilation and cardiovascular collapse
Dicobalt edentate	Binding of cyanide ions by dicobalt edetate and by free cyanide ions	Intravenous injection	Adults: 300 mg (20 mL of 15 mg/mL (15 %) Child: 4–7.5 mg/kg (0.3–0.5 mL/kg of 15 mg/mL (15 %)	50 mL Dextrose (500 g/L) IV immediately after each dose and oxygen	1 min	Urticaria, oedema of face and neck, chest pains, dyspnoea, hypotension, convulsions

(continued)

Table 8.1 (continued)

Therapy	Mechanism	Route	Dose	Concurrent drugs	Admin time	Potential antidote toxicity
Disease mapping and analysis program (DMAP)	Methaemoglobin formation	Intravenous injection	Adults: 3.25 mg/kg Child: 3.25 mg/kg	Oxygen and sodium thiosulphate	1 min	Methaemoglobinaemia, vasodilation and cardiovascular collapse, haemolysis, elevated bilirubin and iron (this is unlikely to be relevant to single dose exposure)
Hydroxocobalamin	Binds cyanide ions	Intravenous injection	Adults: 5–10 g Child: 70 mg/kg	5 g reconstituted in 100 mL 0.9 % saline. Oxygen	20 min	Reddish discoloration to skin and mucous membranes
Sodium thiosulphate	Sulphur donor for endogenous enzymatic conversion of cyanide to thiocyanate	Intravenous injection	Adults: sodium thio-sulphate 25 mL of 500 mg/mL (50 %) solution and oxygen Child: sodium thiosulphate 1.65 mL/kg body weight of 250 mg/mL (25 %) solution (approx. 400 mg/kg body weight) and oxygen	Oxygen and sodium nitrite or Oxygen and DMAP	10 min	Excess administration may cause hypernatraemia

8.3.4   Carbon Monoxide

Carbon monoxide poisoning is a familiar situation in emergency medical practice, and the treatment depends on reversing the attachment of carbon monoxide to haemoglobin as carboxyhaemoglobin using free flow or hyperbaric oxygen therapy. The reader is referred to specialised texts for more details.

8.4   The Management of Lung-Damaging Toxic Trauma

8.4.1   General Considerations

1. Toxic inhalational injury is characteristically different from physical trauma since a clear relationship between cause and effect following a gaseous toxic agent release may be difficult to establish. This is because of the all-important effect of latency of the development of pulmonary damage which has been recognised since the first gas attacks of the First World War. Underlying the management of inhalational toxic injury is the need to keep the patient under careful observation during a potential latent period and to have a very well-tuned index of clinical suspicion that lung damage may be taking place. All through the management of toxic inhalational injury, the importance of latency cannot be over-stated. Awareness of this is a fundamental point of clinical management.
2. Symptoms experienced by the patient such as mild dyspnoea must not be dismissed since they could be of great prognostic importance in the case of inhalational injury.
3. The overall approach to the management of toxic lung injury is not necessarily agent specific. As we have seen, there are many chemical warfare agents and toxic industrial chemicals that can cause pulmonary damage. The important point is that they can be divided into classes of agent that cause damage primarily to the central or to the peripheral compartments of the lung, that is to the upper airways, or the lower peripheral airways and the alveoli. In many cases of inhaled toxic agent injury, the actual identity of the agent release may not be clear. However, whether or not the agent is acting on the central or peripheral compartments of the lung and respiratory tree can be established from a good history and careful examination since the toxidromes are different.

There are few specific therapies available for the management of inhalational injury compared with the management of other toxic trauma (e.g. cyanide and nerve agents). The approach to the management of toxic lung injury must therefore be:

1. Reactive: to deal with potentially life-threatening type 2 respiratory failure with advanced respiratory life-support measures

2. Proactive: to mitigate and pre-empt developing type 1 respiratory failure with the development of toxic pulmonary oedema and acute respiratory distress syndrome during a latent period following exposure.

3. Although there has been a very large amount of experimental work done on toxic pulmonary injury, most of this has been done in animals. Large animal studies, notably in pigs, have produced evidence of the effectiveness of ventilation strategies in proactive management and also of the apparent lack of effectiveness of steroids, for example, in the management of phosgene poisoning. However, the relevance of these studies on man is difficult to assess. The relative rarity of toxic inhalational injury in civil practice (apart from smoke injury) makes the organisation of large-scale human experimental studies to assess the animal results difficult.

4. Where large-scale studies have been organised on the management of lung conditions such as the ARDS group (2000) which can be caused by a wide range of physical and toxic injury, the relevance of the results to the latter remains in question since only a small number of the patients enrolled in the study had toxic inhalation injury as a cause.

5. Equally, there has been a great deal of research into the inflammatory mediators which produce toxic lung injury but so far this has produced little extra in the therapeutic measures available to the clinician.

6. Therefore, the management of toxic inhalational injury is based upon a limited number of airway, ventilation and pharmacological strategies which must be employed in a continuously evolving clinical situation to deal with the developing pathophysiology following toxic inhalational. This is unlike the pathophysiology of cyanide and anticholinesterase poisoning where the injury is produced with short latency and does not (with the exception of intermediate syndrome—see Chap. 9) evolve. The continuous evolution of lung injury has a parallel with the developing longer latency injury of the vesicant agents.

8.4.2   Reactive Treatment

1. In the case of a patient presenting with severe respiratory failure or arrest, immediate life-saving measures will be required. If the patient is still breathing but exhibiting respiratory distress, oxygen therapy with a free flow or demand system (where oxygen supplies may be limited) must be started immediately. Continuing therapy may be with continuous positive airway pressure if the patient is breathing spontaneously. If there is respiratory insufficiency as measured clinically and with blood gas analysis ventilation with positive end-expiratory pressure should be started at once.

2. Bronchospasm

This is an early and important sign of gases that affect the central respiratory compartment (e.g. chlorine). Aggressive treatment is required with bronchodilators (adrenergic agent and theophylline). Steroids should be used if the patient has a history of hyperreactive airways. Steroid doses should be tapered off as rapidly as clinical circumstances permit. Box 8.6 shows details of emergency steroid use following exposure to lung-damaging agents which are discussed further below.

Investigations As soon as the initial surveys are complete and any patient in a life-threatening situation is stabilised, the following baseline and continuing investigations should be carried out:

Chest X-rays (CXRs) and computed tomography (CT) scan (depending on the available facilities—many toxic releases take place in developing nations where resources may be limited). CXR can provide useful information about the development of toxic pulmonary injury. It should be noted, however, that these usually lag behind the developing pathophysiology.

The initial CXR findings after admission may be normal, but as the effects of the exposure continue, there may be bilateral diffuse interstitial infiltrates. An early finding may be hyperinflation indicative of toxic trauma to the smaller airways, resulting in air being trapped in the alveoli.

The appearance of 'batwing' infiltrates indicates the commencement of pulmonary oedema secondary to damage to the alveolar–capillary membrane. Pulmonary oedema develops later without cardiovascular changes of re-distribution or cardiomegaly (Fig. 8.5).

Pulse oximetry This is reliable in the case of pulmonary injury due to lung-damaging agents.

Capnography This is of value in helping to establish a type 2 respiratory failure where end tidal CO_2 characteristically increases.

Arterial blood gases (ABG): The levels of PaO_2 and CO_2 allow the distinction between type 1 and type 2 respiratory failure. In type 1, there is characteristically reduced PaO_2 with normal $PaCO_2$. In type 2, there is reduced PaO_2 with increased $PaCO_2$.

Spirometry (the peak expiratory flow may decrease early after a massive exposure to peripherally acting lung-damaging agents).

Fig. 8.5 Early developing toxic pulmonary oedema. The diffuse opacity in the lung fields is visible only after the effects of developing type 1 respiratory failure

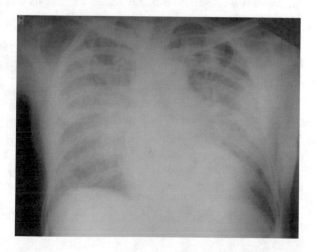

8.4.3 Proactive Treatment

This is required to mitigate as much as possible the effects of the toxic agent in producing acute lung injury, toxic pulmonary oedema and possible ARDS (see Chap. 9).

8.4.3.1 Ventilation Strategy

Early type 2 ventilation failure requires a life-support strategy to clear the airway and start ventilation. The use of a volume preset ventilator is important to ensure the delivery of an adequate tidal volume since there may be decreased compliance (V/P) and increased airway resistance with the development of type 2 respiratory failure.

If there is a developing respiratory failure of the type 1 variety due to acute lung injury and the gradual infiltration of the alveoli, pressure support ventilation may be required. This is normally provided in an intensive care unit as part of a protective ventilation strategy used in the management of ARDS (see Chap. 9).

8.4.3.2 Steroid Therapy

The use of steroids in both the reactive and proactive management of acute toxic lung injury has been the subject of much debate and experimental study. Large animal model studies with phosgene have indicated that the value of steroid therapy in preventing acute lung injury and subsequent toxic pulmonary oedema may only be marginal. However, human studies are lacking, and for this reason, both inhaled and parenteral steroids continue to have a central place in the treatment of all forms of acute lung injury, both physical and toxic. In trauma from lung-damaging agents, they have a clear role in managing the acute bronchospasm which can occur in susceptible individuals. Box 8.6 shows the details of practical steroid therapy for lung-damaging agents.

> **Box 8.6 Emergency steroid therapy following lung-damaging agent exposure**
> If they are to be effective, steroids should be given parenterally as soon as possible after exposure. Once pulmonary oedema has set in, steroids have been shown to be less effective.
>
> A typical regime is methylprednisolone 2000 mg IV or IM at 15 min, 6 and 12 h post-exposure. The dose should be repeated every 12 h for 1–5 days until the risk of developing toxic pulmonary oedema has passed.
>
> Treatment may also be given by steroid inhaler (typically beclomethasone dipropionate) with the initial dose about five times the normal for the

treatment of acute asthma and then half this dose over the next 12 h followed by the standard asthma dose for 72 h or until the risk of pulmonary oedema has passed.

Other drugs that may be useful in the management of the acute phase are:

Aminophylline (bronchospasm)
Salbutamol (bronchospasm)
Codeine phosphate (to suppress cough)

8.4.3.3   Exertion and Toxic Inhalational Injury

During World War I, it was realised early that there was an apparent relationship between poor clinical outcome and exercise during the latent period following exposure to lung-damaging agents such as chlorine and phosgene. The English physiologist John Scott Haldane (Box 8.7) noted clear changes in 'depth of respiration' and prolonged tachycardia after even a mild exercise. This limitation of exercise capability was recognised by field physicians at the time, but the question of whether exercise itself, during the latent period, caused further damage at peripheral lung level remained unresolved.

Box 8.7 John Scott Haldane (1860–1936)

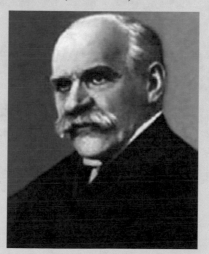

John Scott Haldane (1860–1936) was a distinguished British physiologist who worked on the effects of the first gases used as chemical warfare agents in the First World War. Prior to this, he had studied the suffocative gases occurring in coal mines and made great improvements to safety. At Oxford between 1892 and 1900, Haldane investigated the physiology of the respiration and carriage of oxygen in the blood by haemoglobin. At the request of the War Office, he went to the Western Front in 1915 and identified the gases being used in the first chemical attacks. He developed the first gas mask and also the first field apparatus for oxygen therapy. His contributions to the understanding of the toxic trauma caused by lung-damaging agents remain the basis of therapy to the present day.

At a time when even the most basic of support measures such as the use of oxygen was strictly limited, resting patients who had been exposed to phosgene was one of the things that could be done easily. The problem at the time was the need to discharge exposed casualties back to duty if there was no significant lung damage. The problem still remains for emergency medical responders, dealing with inhalational toxic injury today since, following a mass exposure, there may be limited hospital resources available for admitting patients for bed rest and observation.

Box 8.8 outlines the management of the patient who has been exposed to a lung-damaging agent but who has minimal symptoms at the time of examination.

Box 8.8 Management of exposure to lung-damaging agents but with minimal signs and symptoms
The following points are important to the management of the patient who has been exposed to a lung-damaging agent and who is apparently symptomless, apart from complaining of mild dyspnoea and reduced exercise tolerance:

1. Exercise may cause further harm to the patient and should be restricted until no signs develop during a latent period (the appearance of basal crackles at 4 h is a good indicator of the likelihood of developing toxic pulmonary oedema). Blood gases also provide an early indicator of a developing damage.
2. Oxygen therapy is essential during a latent period, especially if exercise has to be taken.
3. Lung toxic trauma may produce pulmonary abnormalities resulting in dyspnoea. This may not be obvious on initial examination, and it is essential to re-examine the patient at 4–6 h following exposure.
4. Dyspnoea may still be apparent long after CXR, physical examination and ABG have returned to normal. An exercise evaluation of patients complaining of dyspnoea together with ABG analysis is therefore essential.

8.5   The Management of Toxic Trauma from Vesicant Agents

Almost 100 years after the first use of mustard gas (HD) in warfare, there is still no available antidote, although there is an antidote (British anti-Lewisite) to the vesicant Lewisite, an arsenical compound developed in 1919. Treatment is therefore based on early recognition of the exposure and immediate decontamination to prevent further injury. This is particularly important in the case of the eyes.

The previous chapter detailed the toxidrome recognition of exposure to HD. This is based on (1) eye signs, (2) respiratory signs and (3) skin signs.

The eye is the organ most vulnerable to exposure to HD and which requires the earliest possible attention. The signs and symptoms of HD exposure are related to the concentrations of exposure. These concentrations are unlikely to be known to emergency medical responders but are presented in Box 8.9 as an illustration of the dose dependency.

Box 8.9 Effects of specific concentrations of mustard gas

Eyes

(These are usually affected by vapour, and therefore, the toxicity figures are given as concentration × time)

50 mg min m^{-3}: max safe limit of exposure
70 mg min m^{-3}: mild conjunctivitis
100 mg min m^{-3}: partial incapacitation due to eye effects
200 mg min m^{-3}: total incapacitation due to eye effects

NB: In considering vapour exposure, 100 mg min m^{-3} is equivalent to 0.0017 mg/L for 1 h. It should be noted that the odour threshold for HD is 0.0013 mg/L; therefore, there is considerable risk of ocular incapacitation at levels that would be difficult to detect by smell.

Eye signs and symptoms
Low concentration:
Latent period 4–6 h
Lachrymation, burning sensation, pain and visual disturbances
High concentration
Latent period 3–6 h
Conjunctivitis, blepharospasm, photophobia, pain, corneal ulceration

Very high concentrations of HD produce the above toxidrome within a shorter period of 1–2 h depending on the ambient temperature.

Respiratory system
Low concentrations

Nasal irritation, rhinorrhoea, epistaxis, sinus irritation and a burning sensation
in the throat
Latent period 2–4 h
High concentrations
Hoarseness, vocal cord paralysis (aphonia), laryngitis, chest tightness and dry
cough
Latent period 1–3 h
Later: tracheal and bronchial lesions, pseudomembrane production bronchial
obstruction and sloughing—asphyxia

Skin

Liquid exposure
50 mg/cm^2 for 5 min—slight erythema
250–500 mg/cm^2 for 5 min—blistering
(Since much of the exposure will evaporate, it is possible that as little as
6 mg/cm^2 could cause blistering.)
Vapour exposure
100–400 mg min m^{-3}—erythema
200–1000 mg min m^{-3}—blistering
750–1000 mg min m^{-3}—severe incapacitating skin burns
NB: All these effects are greatly enhanced with increased ambient
temperature.

8.5.1   Clinical Management of Mustard Gas Casualties

Key practice points:

1. HD works quickly and causes tissue damage within a few minutes following
   exposure. Thus, removal from exposure and reduction of the effects of the
   remaining contamination by decontamination are of great importance.
2. Decontamination of the eyes must take absolute priority in the early stages of
   management followed by management of the respiratory system. The latency of
   HD and the temperature effects of the toxicity make treatment of the actual
   presenting signs and symptoms difficult.
3. There is no specific treatment for HD in the form of an antidote. Treatment is
   therefore based on early decontamination to reduce further damage, vital
   function life support and management of the skin and other epithelial burns.

8.5.1.1   Eye Management

1. Early decontamination with saline or any other available solution is essential.

   The British CW manual JSP 312 notes that 'attempts to decontaminate the eyes more than 5 min post-exposure are likely to be valueless'.

2. Treat blepharospasm and prevent eye lids from sticking together using Vaseline. Treat eye pain with appropriate anaesthetic drops. Treat photophobia using dark glasses.

8.5.1.2   Essentials of Skin Management

Following an initial erythematous reaction lasting for a few hours post-exposure, small vesicles appear which coalesce to become large vesicles. These are initially painless but become painful with the de-roofing of the vesicles and formation of deep ulcers which can last several months. The Iran–Iraq War (1982–1988) showed that severe HD lesions required several weeks of hospital care followed by prolonged periods of convalescence.

Skin lesions (sometimes called 'chemical burns') can be severe and may appear in extensive areas of the body surface (Fig. 8.6). Naturally, moist areas of the body are most susceptible to HD and crops of blisters may appear at any time up to 2 weeks post-exposure. Box 8.10 summarises aids to treatment for the skin lesions. Much modern experience was gained through the treatment of casualties during the Iran–Iraq War.

(a)   **(b)**

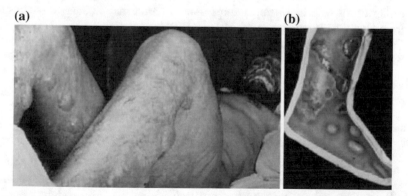

Fig. 8.6 a Vesication of the lower limbs in an Iranian soldier following exposure to sulphur mustard during the Iran–Iraq War. **b** Developing ulceration following the bursting of vesicles caused by sulphur mustard agent. These lesions may take many months to heal and require intensive nursing (*Source* Medical Manual of Defence against Chemical Agents, 6th edition, 1987, HMSO, London)

Box 8.10 Aids to treatment of mustard gas skin lesions

1. Erythema and minor blistering may be treated with Calamine lotion.
2. Silver sulphadiazine was used on Iranian casualties to try to prevent infection.
3. Pain and pruritus (which may be very severe) should be managed by analgesics and antihistamines. Narcotics may be necessary for severe pain.
4. Dilute topical steroids may be beneficial in reducing irritation and oedema at exposed sites. These, however, have little or no effect on the healing of the lesion.
5. Fluid replacement should be calculated using the same regime as for thermal burns.
6. Scars are generally pliable, and contracture is not a major problem.

Note: If the vesicles burst or require de-roofing, the fluid they contain is not a vesicant hazard.

8.5.1.3 Airway and Ventilation Management

1. Observe the patient carefully and regularly for signs of respiratory distress and failure. These must be treated immediately for other classes of toxic hazard.
2. Observe the breathing: rate, form, depth as described for the management of other toxic agents. Respiratory distress in HD exposure develops with a longer latency than other agents affecting the respiratory system. The appearance of respiratory problems is dependent on the ambient temperature. There is an earlier onset with high temperatures. Auscultation may indicate bronchospasm from chemical bronchiolitis.
   Cough and expectoration feature after a few hours following exposure.
3. Airway clearance and management.

This should follow the guidelines for early life support given above.

8.6 Management of Exposure to Riot Control Agents

Riot control agents sometimes called primary chemosensory irritant chemicals (PCSI) such as 2-chlorobenzalmalononitrile (CS) gas are used widely around the world by police forces. Riot control agents have an immediate and disabling effect due to their actions on the eyes and upper respiratory system. However, the safety margin between the effective and lethal doses is one of the largest for any chemical agent. This has been established by extensive research, and as a result, riot control agents are not classed as chemical warfare agents by the 1992 Chemical Warfare Convention. They do not cause any lasting respiratory distress or consequences but the immediate actions are very distressing and off-gassing of patients who may have contaminated clothing can cause secondary effects in the emergency room.

Treatment of mild exposure to CS gas is usually not necessary apart from reassurance. If there has been a severe exposure (e.g. in a patient who was close to the canister when discharged), the following actions should be taken:

1. Eyes

   Contamination of the eyes by liquid agent should be removed by irrigating immediately with normal saline. Pain should be treated with anaesthetic eye drops. Blepharitis may occur and should be treated with tetracaine ointment. An ophthalmological opinion should be sought for serious cases.

2. Skin

   The skin should be decontaminated with soap and water. Any local erythema will resolve within hours. Occasionally, there may be exposure to solid CS which can cause vesication. This should be treated using conventional burn protocols.

3. Respiratory system

   Upper respiratory symptoms and cough usually resolve rapidly following exposure. Bronchitis may occur in some cases and should be treated conventionally.

Other riot control agents exist but are not so widely used as CS gas (e.g. dibenzoxazepine, CR). The management principles are essentially the same as for CS but CR is more persistent and may pose a hazard to hospital responders. The reader is referred to specialised texts for more information.

8.7   Conclusions

In the management of toxic trauma, the provision of early life-support measures must take priority for cases which are triaged as requiring immediate care. A wide range of severity of injury is likely depending on the degree of exposure and should be treated appropriately, with consideration of the potential risks and benefit in the case of some antidotes. Antidotes exist for relatively few toxic agents but there are a number of supportive treatment options available which are summarised in this chapter. More detail can be found in the specialised texts listed in the suggestions for further reading.

Further Reading

Baskin SJ, Kelly JB, Maliner BI et al (2008) Cyanide poisoning. In: Tuorinsky SD (ed) Medical aspects of chemical warfare, Chap. 11. Office of the Surgeon General, United States Army Borden Institute, Walter Reed Army Medical Center, Washington DC, pp 371–410

Eyer PA, Worek F (2007) Oximes. In: Marrs TC, Maynard RL, Sidell FR (eds) Chemical warfare agents; toxicology and treatment, 2nd edn. Wiley, Chichester

Hurst CG, Petrali JP, Barillo DJ (2008) Vesicants. In: Tuorinsky SD (ed) Medical aspects of chemical warfare, Chap. 8. Office of the Surgeon General, United States Army Borden Institute, Walter Reed Army Medical Center, Washington DC, pp 259–307

Marrs T, Rice P, Vale A (2006) The role of oximes in the treatment of nerve agent poisoning in civilan casualties. Toxicol Rev 25(4):297–323

Marrs TC, Maynard RL, Sidell FR (2007) Chemical warfare agents: toxicology and treatment. Wiley, Chichester

Ministry of Defence (1987) Medical manual of defence against chemical agents (JSP 312). Her Majesty's Stationery Office, London

Sidell FR, Newmark J, McDonough JH (2008) Nerve agents. In Tuorinsky SD (ed) Medical aspects of chemical warfare, Chap. 5. Office of the Surgeon General, United States Army Borden Institute, Walter Reed Army Medical Center, Washington DC, pp 155–242

Tuorinsky SD, Sciuto AM (2008) Toxic inhalation injury and toxic industrial chemicals. In: Tuorinsky SD (ed) Medical aspects of chemical and biological warfare, Chap. 10. Office of the Surgeon General, United States Army, Borden Institure, Walter Reed Army Center, Washington DC, pp 339–370

Wattana M, Bey T (2009) Mustard gas or sulphur mustard: an old chemical agents as new terrorist threat. Prehosp Disaster Med 24(1):19–29

Willems JL (1989) Clinical management of mustard gas casualties. Ann Med Milit Belg 3(suppl):1

Chapter 9
The Longer-Term Consequences of Toxic Trauma

Abstract The period up to 24 h following the emergency management of acute toxic exposure is of critical importance in the prevention and recognition of developing pathology with a longer latency. The nervous system may develop a re-paralysis following the depolarising paralysis of the acute cholinergic system. This re-paralysis is a non-depolarising block, known as intermediate syndrome and may indicate a conformational change in the acetylcholine receptors in the neuro-muscular junction leading to a failure of transmission and subsequent muscle paralysis. After a week following exposure to organophosphate (OP) pesticides, the peripheral nervous system may also develop OP-induced delayed neuropathy (OIPDN). In the lungs, toxic pulmonary oedema may develop after 12–24 h following exposure to lung-damaging agents. Resting a patient at risk, using steroids and applying appropriate protective artificial ventilation measures may modify the onset of pulmonary oedema and possibly acute respiratory distress syndrome.

9.1 Introduction

As we have seen in the previous chapters, exposure to toxic chemical agents produces effects after a short-time span which requires urgent emergency intervention in both the pre-hospital and hospital emergency room settings. However, post-acute management of toxic trauma in a hospital can last days or weeks. In addition, there may be developing conditions which are either related to the initial presentation or are a result of long-latency toxicity of the causative agent.

Many toxic substances, if not lethal in the first instance, have considerable long-term effects lasting for many years in some cases. This was realised after the First World War when there were a large number of disability pensions issued for the effects of mainly lung-damaging agents and vesicants. In civil life too, there are well-documented long-term effects of acute exposures to toxic agents, apart from the effects of chronic exposure such as the methyl isocyanate release at Bhopal where related respiratory conditions are still being treated today (see Chap. 10).

Such long-term consequences of toxic trauma can place a considerable burden on health services, particularly in poorer parts of the world where medical resources are limited.

The many long-term diseases caused by exposure to toxic chemical agents are managed by a range of specialties, and the details are outside the scope of this book. This chapter considers briefly the longer-term sequelae of acute toxic trauma in relation to early emergency care and how this may affect the development of conditions appearing with longer latency.

9.2   Central Nervous System

9.2.1   Organophosphates

Long-term central nervous effects, following both acute and chronic exposures to organophosphate (OP) toxic agents, have been reported for many years and include inability to concentrate, sleep disorders and persistent dreaming. In addition, there was evidence of similar effects in chronic low-level exposure to OP agents among sarin workers in the early 1970s. These persisting CNS effects were of considerable interest to the military during the Cold War as they would lead to significant degradation among specially trained members of the forces which would make them unfit for duty and place a considerable strain on the military medical care systems.

In addition to the milder long-term effects of OPs, there may be central effects as a result of the hypoxia that may have occurred during convulsions and possible respiratory insufficiency during an acute cholinergic syndrome.

9.2.2   Incapacitating Agents

Incapacitating agents such as lysergic acid diethylamide (LSD) and 3-quinuclidinyl benzilate (BZ) have extended acute effects of confusion and delirium. Recovery is usually complete in the case of BZ exposure following rest and psychiatric support in some cases. Following studies in the 1960s, LSD was known to cause long-term psychotic effects in certain persons who appeared to have individual susceptibility. It also had widely unpredictable actions in subjects tested and was therefore not considered by the military as a viable incapacitating agent.

Opioid-incapacitating agents may cause prolonged respiratory depression, but recovery is usually without sequelae after a period of artificial ventilation and the administration of repeated doses of naloxone.

9.3 Peripheral Nervous System

9.3.1 Development of the Acute Cholinergic Syndrome

The presentation and initial treatment of the characteristic acute cholinergic syndrome following severe OP exposure was considered in earlier chapters. Experience with OP pesticide poisoning has shown that in most cases, the signs and symptoms resolve after about 18 h with continuing anticholinergic and oxime treatment. Ventilation, if it had been required, can be discontinued at this stage.

Experience with nerve agents is more limited. In the case of some nerve agents, such as soman (GD), which quickly produce an irreversible complex with acetylcholinesterase, an extension of the cholinergic period may be expected with appropriate life support if there is significant respiratory failure.

9.3.2 Intermediate Syndrome

The OP-induced intermediate syndrome (IMS) presents a pathophysiological development which has important consequences for subsequent critical care management. In a study of patients treated for ingestion of OP pesticides, the neurologist Nimal Sennanayake and the anaesthesiologist Lakshman Karralliede, working in Sri Lanka in 1987, described a re-paralysis of 10–20 % of patients who had been admitted for acute OP pesticide poisoning at 18–24 h following resolution of the acute cholinergic syndrome which had been severe enough to require ventilation and atropine and pralidoxime treatment. The condition they encountered was a gradual re-paralysis of proximal and respiratory muscles which was characterised initially by an inability to lift the head off a pillow (a standard basic anaesthetic test to assess reversal of the actions of a non-depolarising muscle relaxant following general anaesthesia).

When re-paralysis occurred in these patients, it was different from the classic depolarisation paralysis of the acute cholinergic syndrome. Repetitive nerve stimulation of muscles showed decrementing responses, signifying the development of a non-depolarising block of the type produced by muscle relaxants used in general anaesthesia such as curare and vecuronium. In acute cholinergic paralysis, repeated stimulation of muscle shows a diminished but non-decrementing response. This is seen after the administration of the short-acting muscle relaxant succinylcholine (which chemically is two molecules of acetylcholine joined together).

After re-paralysis occurred, artificial ventilation was required for extended periods of several days. The syndrome was confirmed by many authors during the 1990s. It was later realised that a similar condition had been described by R. S. Wadia in India in the 1970s who called the depolarising and non-depolarising blocks phases I and II, respectively. Another condition, described in general anaesthesia in the 1960s which closely mimics IMS, is known as dual block. This is the development of a non-depolarising block following repeated doses of the depolarising neuromuscular-blocking agent succinylcholine where a non-depolarising block occurred. There are also similarities with myasthenia gravis where there is an immune-based downregulation (reduction in density of AChR at the post-junctional membrane).

Clinical neurophysiological studies of IMS have indicated fade at low-frequency stimulation and the absence of post-tetanic facilitation which points to a post-junctional lesion. More experimental information has been provided from single fibre electromyography (SFEMG), a sensitive neurophysiological technique which can detect failure of acetylcholine receptors on muscle fibres long before clinical weakness is noted. This technique analyses the small time differences between muscle fibre action potentials in a motor unit (a group of muscle fibres innervated by a single motor neurone). The time variation, known as jitter, is directly linked to the security of neuromuscular transmission. Box 9.1 and Figs 9.1 and 9.2 give details.

Box 9.1 SFEMG jitter following OP exposure

Single fibre electromyography (SFEMG) is a sensitive clinical neurophysiological technique used to assess failure of nerve impulse transmission at the neuromuscular junction (NMJ). SFEMG records the time variations (jitter) between two muscle fibre action potentials from fibres activated by a common terminal nerve fibre. The action potentials are recorded with a very small electrode placed between two fibres in a muscle being activated either by voluntarily or by electrical stimulation from a second electrode. Jitter can be observed and measured by displaying the signals on an oscilloscope where there is a variation in the interpotential interval (Figs. 9.1 and 9.2).

The degree of recorded jitter in SFEMG is directly related to the release of ACh and the function of the ACh receptors in the NMJ. SFEMG therefore provides a window into the operation of the NMJ. Jitter is characteristically increased in conditions (both pre- and post-junctional) of the NMJ which reduce the safety margins of neuromuscular transmission. Thus, there is increased jitter in conditions such as myasthenia gravis and Lambert–Eaton syndrome. Jitter is also increased following the administration of small doses

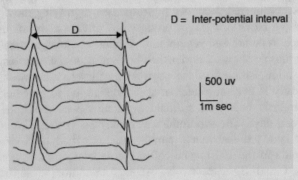

D = Inter-potential interval

500 uv

1m sec

Fig. 9.1 Muscle fibre action potentials from a motor unit displayed sequentially. The firing rate is 15 Hz

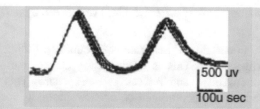

Fig. 9.2 Ten superimposed sweeps from the sequential display showing the jitter of the second action potential showing time variation, or jitter in the appearance of the second action potential. (*Source* Author's original recordings)

of muscle relaxants and low doses of the organophosphate anticholinesterase sarin. Single fibre electromyography is very sensitive and is able to detect alternations in neuromuscular transmission before any clinical muscle weakness is apparent and before any fade of the overall muscle response to stimulation can be detected.

The Eaton–Lambert syndrome and administration of small doses of non-depolarising muscle blockers such as curare cause jitter increases and in some cases lead to a failure of firing of muscle fibres, known as blocking. Significant degrees of blocking are detected as fade, following conventional repetitive stimulation, but SFEMG will detect changes in neuromuscular transmission long before they are evident using conventional techniques and clinical observation. In 1996, Baker and Sedgwick reported an SFEMG study of eight fit volunteers exposed to trace amounts of sarin sufficient to cause miosis and a sensation of tightness in the chest but with no other signs or symptoms. The study showed small increased jitter changes after exposure which resolved within 1 year. These results may indicate a subclinical change in neuromuscular (NM) safety margin after non-toxic OP exposure.

Both peripheral neuropathy and myopathy (vide infra) have been suggested as the basis of the pathophysiology of IMS, but current available evidence suggests that the neuromuscular junction (NMJ) is the critical site. At the present time, experimental and clinical evidence suggest that following prolonged depolarising block, the structure of the acetylcholine receptors in the NMJ is altered leading to a gradual failure of transmission and consequent muscle paralysis.

9.3.2.1 Management of IMS

Clinically, IMS resembles the syndrome of incomplete reversal of neuromuscular paralysis by non-depolarising blocking agents sometimes seen following general anaesthesia. Patients will recover after a week or 10 days if intensive care facilities are available with intermediate positive pressure variation. Unfortunately, OP pesticide poisoning often occurs in countries that have the least available resources in terms of intensive care.

9.3.3   Organophosphate-Induced Delayed Neuropathy

Following exposure to certain OP pesticide compounds, a further long-term complication has been described. This is OP-induced delayed neuropathy (OPIDN) which can appear between 1 and 3 weeks post-exposure. This peripheral neuropathy is characterised by incoordination, ataxia, spasticity and flaccid muscle paralysis. Unlike IMS, the condition begins in the lower limbs and then spreads to the upper limbs. In severe cases, the result may be permanent quadriplegia.

The condition has been shown histopathologically to be associated with changes at the distal section of a peripheral motor nerve with progressive demyelination. This is characterised by a reduction in nerve conduction velocity in clinical neurophysiological studies.

OPIDN is thought to be mediated by OP acting not as an anticholinesterase but as a neurotoxic esterase. The condition is not seen in poisonings by all OP pesticides and has not yet been reported in humans exposed to nerve gases.

However, there are large differences between the databases of OP pesticide exposure and nerve agent exposure in humans. One report from the 1995 Tokyo sarin release concerned a patient who survived for 15 months following the attack and then showed signs of a distal sensory neuropathy. However, since he was on life support for much of this time, there is no clear link with sarin as a cause.

In addition to OPIDN, in experimental animal studies, OP compounds have been shown to be associated with muscle necrosis in the region of the end plate of the NMJ. The clinical significance of this finding in humans remains unclear.

9.4   Longer-Term Effects of Toxic Agent Exposure on the Respiratory System

The period up to 24 h following the acute upper respiratory effects of inhalation of irritant lung-damaging agents is of great importance in managing and particularly in preventing toxic pulmonary oedema (PE) which may lead to the onset of acute respiratory distress syndrome. As noted previously, any patient who is at risk of developing PE should be carefully observed over a 24-h period, preferably with bed rest. Following mass exposure, this will place a considerable strain on medical resources. This emphasises the importance of accurate clinical triage and assessment following admission and of continued assessment during the latent period leading up to secondary effects. Apart from bed rest and the normal management of early respiratory signs and symptoms such as cough and bronchospasm, management of developing lung problems depends largely on the use of steroids and an appropriate ventilation strategy for those at risk.

9.4.1 Management of Toxic Pulmonary Oedema

9.4.1.1 The Use of Steroids

There has been considerable debate about the rationale for the use of systemic and inhaled steroids in the treatment of toxic PE. Theoretically, there should be many advantages such as the inhibition of phospholipase A_2 via induced lipomodulin and macrocortin, inhibition of macrophages, inhibition of the production of prostanoids and leukotrienes and stimulation of surfactant production in type II cells. However, beneficial effects only follow early administration while late administration may be deleterious (inhibition of production of type I cells and enhanced fibroblast production). More recently, studies have been published on animal models. A number of studies on pigs have shown variable results including one where inhaled beclomethasone showed improved PaO_2, improved ventilation to perfusion ratio and less histological damage. However, species differences exist, and results should be applied with caution to humans.

The acute lung injury group in 2002, reviewing the effects of steroid therapy on the prevention of acute respiratory distress syndrome (ARDS) from all causes, concluded that there was no proven case for their use. However, it should be noted that because toxic lung injury is rare compared to the other causes of ARDS, the number of respiratory toxic trauma cases included in the study was low. Therefore, at present, although the use of steroids in preventing respiratory complications in animal models has indicated limited benefit, withholding their use in humans remains unproven. At the present time, therefore, the use of inhaled steroids for developing toxic PE in humans should not be discounted, particularly in view of the limited therapeutic options available.

9.4.1.2 Ventilation and Developing Toxic Pulmonary Oedema

The timing and technique of artificial ventilation may have important consequences for the management of development of toxic PE. In particular, the early use of a bag-valve mask (BVM) ventilation may have deleterious effect on damaged alveolar tissue. It is known that automatic ventilation from portable emergency ventilators provides more accurate ventilation in the field than BVM techniques (Baker 2016). Poorly controlled emergency ventilation may cause alveolar wall damage as well as barotraumas. It is now well established that inappropriate ventilation in the intensive care unit may provoke ARDS due to kinin release due to repeated opening and closing of alveoli. This has lead to the 'open lung' strategy of pressure support ventilation where collapsed alveoli are opened and then kept open by application of positive end-expiratory pressure (PEEP) and low-tidal volumes. This technique may have an application in the early management of patients who are at risk of developing toxic PE. Management of developing toxic PE provides a major ventilatory challenge even in a sophisticated modern intensive care unit (ICU) where all ventilatory modes are available. Patients who have been exposed to oedemagens but have not yet showed any signs or symptoms of developing PE should be confined to bed and observed for at least 24 h, if possible.

9.5   Long-Term Respiratory Conditions Following Exposure to Lung-Damaging Agents

The large number of casualties from chlorine and phosgene exposure during World War I showed that survivors showed long-term respiratory disorders with chronic bronchitis and emphysema, the most common conditions, followed by pulmonary fibrosis. The Bhopal incident in India (see Chap. 10) has also shown evidence of long-term respiratory disorders following exposure to the toxic industrial pulmonary oedemagen methyl isocyanate.

9.6   Long-Term Effects of Exposure to Mustard Gas

Information about the long-term effects of exposure to mustard gas comes from two major sources separated by almost a century. As with lung-damaging agents, there was a study of the long-term effects of mustard gas casualties in World War I, some of whom died as a direct result of the effects of the exposure some years later. The Iran–Iraq War during the 1980s provided an opportunity to study a large number of survivors of mustard gas exposure using modern techniques. The US Veterans Administration conducted a study in 1993 which showed a causal relationship between exposure to mustard gas and a wide range of conditions including chronic respiratory diseases (asthma, chronic bronchitis, emphysema, chronic obstructive airway disease and chronic laryngitis), carcinomas of the respiratory tract, skin pigmentation abnormalities and neoplasms, bone marrow depression, eye conditions including chronic conjunctivitis, recurrent corneal ulceration and delayed recurrent keratitis. In addition, psychological disorders were reported including mood and anxiety disorders which had also been noted following the First World War.

A follow-up study of 200 Iranian soldiers who had received severe injuries from mustard gas during the Iran–Iraq War showed that about one-third had persistent respiratory effects two years following exposure notably chronic bronchitis, asthma, tracheobronchitis, laryngitis, recurrent pneumonia and bronchiectasis. Those who had suffered a high concentration exposure to the large airways developed tracheobronchial stenosis.

9.7 Conclusions

There are established long-term sequelae following acute exposure to a number of toxic agents, both chemical warfare and toxic industrial chemicals. The management of these is covered by a number of medical specialities but emergency responders to toxic trauma should be aware of the longer-term consequences when applying emergency medical care both at the time of the exposure and in the period immediately afterwards. For respiratory conditions, proactive measures such as pharmacological intervention and ventilation strategies can affect the outcome. The long-term eye conditions following mustard gas exposure underline the importance of immediate decontamination and early ocular care.

Further Reading

Baker DJ (2016) Artificial ventilation: a basic clinical guide. Springer, London

Baker DJ (2005) Critical care requirements after mass toxic agent release. Crit Care Med 33: S66–74

Baker DJ, Sedgwick ME (1996) Single fibre electromyographic changes after OP exposure. Hum Exp Toxicol 15:369–337

Balali-Mood M (1986) First report of delayed toxic effect of Yperite poisoning in Iranian fighters. In: Proceedings of the 2nd world congress on new compounds in biological and chemical warfare: toxicological evaluation, industrial chemical disasters, civil protection and treatment. International Association of Forensic Toxicologists, Ghent, 24–27 Aug 1986, pp 489–495

Karalliedde L, Baker DJ, Marrs T (2006a) Organophosphate—induced intermediate syndrome: etiology and relationships with myopathy. Toxicol Rev 25(1):1–14

Karalliedde L., Baker DJ, Marrs TC (2006b) OP-Induced Intermediate Syndrome: aetiology and relationships with myopathy. Toxicol Rev 25:1176–2551

Ketchum JS, Salem H (2007) Incapacitating agents. In: Tuorinsky SD (ed) Medical aspects of chemical and biological warfare. Borden Institute. Office of the Surgeon General, pp 411–439 (Chap. 12)

Parkhouse DA, Brown RFR, Jugg BJA et al (2007) Protective ventilation strategy in the management of phosgene—induced acute lung injury. Mil Med 172:295–300

Papadakos P, Lachmann B (2002) The open lung concept of alveolar recruitment can improve outcome in respiratory failure and ARDS. Mt Sinai J Med 69(1–2):73

Pechura CM, Rall DP (eds) (1993) Veterans at risk: the health effects of mustard gas and Lewisite. National Academy Press, Washington, DC

Reis MD, Gommers D, Lachmann B (2008) Open lung management. In: Papadakos PP, Lachman B (eds) Mechanical ventilation: clinical applications and pathophysiology. Sanders—Elsevier, Philadelphia, pp 276–285 (Chap. 25)

Senanayake N, Karalliedde L (1987) Neurotoxic effects of organophosphorus insecticides: an intermediate syndrome. N Eng J Med 316(13):761–763

Smith WJ, Clark MG, Talbot TB et al (2007) Long term health effects of chemical threat agents. In: Tuorinsky SD (ed) Medical aspects of chemical and biological warfare. Borden Institute. Office of the Surgeon General, pp 311–337 (Chap. 9)

Smith WJ, Clark MG, Talbot TB (2008) Longer term health effects of chemical threat agents. In: Tuorinsky SD (ed) Medical aspects of chemical and biological warfare. Office of the Surgeon General, United States Army, Borden Institute, Walter Reed Army Center, Washington, DC, pp 339–370 (Chap 10)

The Acute Respiratory Distress Syndrome Network (2000) Ventilation with lower tidal volumes as
    compared with traditional tidal volumes for acute lung injury and the respiratory distress
    syndrome. N Eng J Med 342(18):1301–1308
Varma DR, Guest I (1993) The Bhopal incident and methyl isocyanate toxicity. J Toxicol Environ
    Health 40:513–529
Willems JL (1989) Clinical management of mustard gas casualties. Ann Med Milit Belg 3(suppl
    1):1–61
Wheeler AP, Barnard GR (2007) Acute lung injury and the acute respitory distress syndrome: a
    clinical review. Lancet 335:1553–1565
Zaimis E, Head S (1976) Depolarizing neuromuscular blocking drugs. In: Handbook of
    experimental pharmacology: 42 the neuromuscular junction. Springer, Berlin (Chap. 4a)

Chapter 10
Preparing for Toxic Trauma

Abstract Awareness and preparation by emergency medical responders for possible mass casualties from a toxic chemical release is an essential part of disaster response. Although individual poisoning and small-scale chemical incidents occur on a regular basis, large-scale releases are relatively uncommon and medical experience in managing casualties with toxic trauma is limited. A number of major chemical releases that have taken place over the past 100 years are considered in this chapter. These provide many lessons for those preparing for the management of toxic trauma. In addition, for planning a response, individual training, particularly in protection and application of medical knowledge from common medical conditions that mimic the effects of chemical agents, such as asthma and acute lung injury, all contribute to building an effective response to mass chemical casualties, an occurrence, we must hope, will continue to be a rarity.

10.1 Introduction

Large-scale chemical releases are rare events around the world. Thus, direct emergency medical experience of dealing with toxic trauma is relatively limited compared with physical trauma, which occurs on a daily basis. However, the risk of both accidental and deliberate toxic releases is growing and emergency medical teams must plan, prepare and train for such events. To do this, the following are required:

1. Awareness of the risks involved.
2. Learning the lessons from previous toxic disasters.
3. Applying medical experience in the management of illnesses that have features that are analogous to those of toxic trauma.

© Springer International Publishing Switzerland 2016
D.J. Baker, *Toxic Trauma*, DOI 10.1007/978-3-319-40916-0_10

10.2   The Risk of a Toxic Chemical Agent Release

Toxic chemical agents while in containers pose no immediate hazard to those in the vicinity. When released from the container, however, the contained hazard poses a risk. Risk is defined essentially as the probability of a hazard occurring. The risks of an accidental or deliberate chemical release are difficult to quantify precisely but are probably increasing in both the developed and developing nations. In the UK alone, 70,000 chemicals are used industrially, more than 2000 of which are considered harmful toxic industrial chemicals (TICs). A total of 200,000 t is transported daily. Although the Control of Major Accident Hazard (COMAH) 1999 Regulations (amended in 2005) were designed to reduce the risk to the public from harmful releases from large chemical and related industries, there are many companies which are too small to be subject to these regulations.

Within emergency medicine, it is a common perception that chemical incidents are rare events. It has often been quoted in the past that there are approximately 1000 acute chemical incidents per year in England and Wales that may impact human health and that the majority of these events involve less than four casualties. For the purposes of public health, a chemical incident is defined as 'an event in which there is, or could be, exposure of the public to chemical substances that cause, or have the potential to cause, ill health'. Hospital staff and emergency services personnel are considered to be members of the public in this definition. In 2005, the UK Health Protection Agency recorded more than 1000 chemical incidents, and it was estimated that approximately 27,000 people may have been exposed, of whom about 3000 reported with symptoms. It is thought that the actual numbers may be considerably higher.

Worldwide, industrial accidents that involve an extremely large number of casualties resulting from chemical exposures are rare. Between 1975 and 1999, 25 incidents involving more than 25 fatalities and 100 injured were recorded.

In the civil setting, the deliberate release of chemicals has also occurred. The series of deliberate chemical releases in Japan in the 1990s, most notably the sarin attacks in Matsumoto in 1994 and on the Tokyo subway network in 1995, showed that even relatively small terrorist groups have the capability to produce and deploy chemical weapons. In addition, the targeting of a road chlorine tanker in Iraq in 2006 by terrorists has emphasised that improvised explosive devices may be used by terrorists to disseminate toxic agents explosively and thus create casualties with both physical and toxic trauma.

10.3   Key Medical Lessons Learned from Previous Releases of Toxic Chemical Agents

The major releases of toxic chemical agents in both war and peace over the past 100 years have provided medical lessons, which are of value to all those involved in both planning and response to toxic releases. This section considers some important examples.

10.3.1   World War I

1. As noted in Chap. 2, the first large-scale chemical attack in 1915 was totally unexpected and the targets were unprotected. Very heavy casualties were suffered from the high concentrations of chlorine achieved in Allied trenches due to a mass-synchronised release of chlorine from cylinders in the German trenches. The rapid onset of both upper and lower respiratory tract effects highlights the limitation of the Haber principle at high concentrations. There were early choking upper respiratory effects and also early evidence of toxic pulmonary oedema (with a latency considerably less than the usual 18–24 h).
2. Following the early attacks, protective masks were rapidly developed and the subsequent mortality rates were relatively low compared with the first attack. This highlights the importance of personal protection in mitigating the effects of a toxic agent release.
3. At the time of the 1915 attacks and throughout the remainder of the First World War, respiratory life support was unknown, and the management of toxic pulmonary oedema was ineffective (with the exception of the recognition of the importance of resting after a phosgene attack to reduce pulmonary arterial pressure as much as possible).
4. The use of phosgene gas by both sides continued for the rest of the war and caused the most fatalities from chemical warfare agents. Because of its lower water solubility compared with chlorine, phosgene was found to be more effective in producing a late onset of pulmonary oedema at lower concentrations. It was therefore more toxic than chlorine. It also caused immediate incapacitation due to its short latency upper respiratory tract actions ('irritant' or 'choking').
   The key lesson was the importance of the development of toxic pulmonary oedema from exposure to lung-damaging agents.
5. Hydrogen cyanide was used by the French Army with limited effect due to its non-persistent characteristics. This illustrates the importance of the physical properties of a released toxic chemical agent and the prevailing weather conditions and is a good example of the importance of persistence as one of the many factors contributing to the development of toxic trauma.

6. The year 1917 saw the first German use of sulphur mustard gas which had originally been considered as a chemical warfare agent by the British but was discounted. Mustard gas was the first chemical warfare agent with a long latency to be used essentially to disable fighting men (i.e. to wound rather than to kill). The key lesson from the first and subsequent use of mustard gas is the danger of a persistent agent to responders and the long-term incapacitating effects on those exposed (see Chap. 9).

10.3.2   1936: Italian Use of Mustard Gas in Abyssinia

In 1936, in Abyssinia, the Italian Army used mustard gas systematically against totally unprotected civilian targets who suffered heavy casualties with little or no medical care. This was the first use of a chemical warfare agent against a civilian population and led to major preparations being made on both sides, during the beginning of the Second World War, to protect cities against gas attacks. In the event, no gas attacks took place in Europe although there were some in the war between Japan and China in Manchuria.

10.3.3   Use of Nerve Agents and Mustard Gas in the Iran–Iraq War

The Iran–Iraq war provided the first wartime casualties from the use of nerve agents who were documented and treated by well-trained physicians using modern equipment. The use of modern antidotes and life support measures kept the mortality low. Personal protective equipment was available but there was a failure of protection with filtration respirators due to the fact that many of the soldiers had beards. The low dead-to-wounded ratio (<2 %) reflected the immediate and continuing respiratory and antidote care provided.

10.3.4   Chemical Attack Against Civilians in Hallabja, Kurdistan

Hallabja is a small town about 150 miles north-east of Baghdad and is close to the Iranian border. On 16 March 1988, the Iraqi Army launched a chemical attack on the civilian population to halt the Iranian advance and also to attack a Kurdish minority. The aerial attack started with high explosive bombs following which the planes dropped 10 L canisters containing what is thought to be a cocktail of chemical warfare agents, designed to confuse diagnosis in those affected. The information about the attack comes largely from survivors who described the canister bombs falling with a muffled thump, following which white clouds were released, smelling of garlic and sweet apples. There is still confusion about exactly which chemical agents were used, but the fatalities were produced with a very short latency. Eyewitness accounts following the attack described dead bodies in the streets, at the steering wheels of their cars and huddled in doorways (Fig. 10.1). The skin of the bodies was noticed to be strangely discoloured, and the eyes of the victims were open and staring. This attack was the first confirmed large-scale chemical attack on civilians, and the results show the devastation that may be caused when chemical weapons are used against unprotected and untrained civilians with little or no immediate emergency medical aid.

A number of questions about the attack at Hallabja remain unanswered to this day:

1. No fragments of chemical munitions were found. The site was presumed to have been cleared by Iraqi or Iranian troops.
2. The photographs published after the incident gave an impression that the dead had been arranged to create a more horrific impression.
3. Some victims were noted to have bright blue lips raising the question about whether hydrogen cyanide had been included in the chemical munition. This is an impurity in the nerve gas tabun (GA). Intelligence has shown that the Iraqi Army had the capability to produce this nerve agent and sarin together with sulphur mustard gas.

Following the attack, the non-governmental organisation, Physicians for Human Rights sent an investigating team to Hallabja to question survivors. They confirmed attacks by low-flying aircraft and the bursting of chemical munitions. The investigators concluded that the attack had been carried out using mustard gas mixed with at least one type of nerve agent.

The attack on Hallabja highlights the effects of a chemical attack on an unprotected population with little or no awareness. It reinforced the public viewpoint that chemical weapons are essentially weapons of mass destruction and that

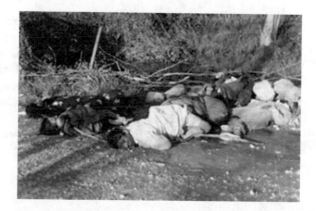

Fig. 10.1 Fatalities from the Iraqi chemical attack on Halabja, March 1988 (*Source* The Kurdish Observer, 16/03/12)

little can be done for those exposed. In reality, if the population in Hallabja had been provided with even a basic personal protection, such as the gas masks issued in Europe at the beginning of the Second World War, the level of fatalities would have been very different. The relatively low fatality rate from chemical exposure in the Iranian Army during the Iran–Iraq war and the availability of early life support and antidote treatment illustrates this point.

10.3.5   1994–1995: Terrorist Sarin Attacks in Matsumoto and Tokyo, Japan

10.3.5.1   Matsumoto

On 27 June 1994, the first successful terrorist attack on a civil population took place in the Japanese city of Matsumoto in the northern Japanese mountains. It was carried out by a cult (Aum Shinrikyo) that had managed to synthesise sarin in a secret laboratory and released it at night from a van. The attack resulted in 600 casualties and seven fatalities. Five of these were found dead, and two were transported to the hospital where one died of respiratory failure and secondary cardiac arrest within 4 h and the other died many years later after having been in a vegetative state. Fifty-six persons were hospitalised in six hospitals. Respiratory failure was evident from the outset, and several casualties required intubation and ventilation. Generalised convulsions were noted in a number of cases. Not all the persons affected required hospital treatment, with some seeking medical evaluation later and other symptomatic cases which did not require medical care.

The attack was revealed only after 2 h by a telephone call for emergency medical care. Eight of the medical responders including one doctor suffered anticholinergic effects as a result of cross-contamination.

10.3.5.2   Tokyo Metro Sarin Attack

On 20 March 1995, Aum Shinrikyo launched a further sarin attack, this time on the Tokyo underground railway system. About 24 litres of sarin of only 30 % purity were released from polythene carrier bags by cult members.

The attack involved five different underground trains, all of which were scheduled to arrive between 0800 and 0810 h on Kasumigaseki station, close to the Tokyo National Police Agency and the Japanese Finance Ministry. The city fire department, who have responsibility for toxic agent releases, was informed within 15 min of the attack which in the event involved 15 metro stations. The hospitals in the area were notified that there had been a gas explosion and were prepared to receive patients with burns, blast injury and carbon monoxide poisoning. The confusion about the nature of the event remained for nearly an hour during which

131 ambulances and more than 1000 ambulance personnel were sent to the stations affected. As a result of encouragement by the media and problems with communication with the emergency operations centre, most of the casualties were transported to the closest hospital, St. Luke's International Hospital. As a result, this hospital saw nearly 650 casualties within the first 24 h after the release.

The agent used in the attack was not recognised until about 2.5 h after the attack when the classic nerve agent toxidrome was recognised by physicians who had attended the patients in the Matsumoto attack.

The emergency medical technicians (EMT) who arrived at the site of the release carried out triage of patients, but there was no respiratory life support or administration of antidotes. Because the EMT had no protective equipment, some 135 of them became secondary casualties, of which 25 required hospitalisation.

At St. Luke's, there was no attempt at securing the emergency department and there was full access by television crews and onlookers. Twenty-three per cent of the staff in the emergency department themselves experienced mild nerve agent symptoms which were enough to interfere with their working ability.

The attack resulted in 12 fatalities, six of which occurred within 2 h of the release and 6 between 20 and 80 days later. At St Luke's, two deaths resulted from cardiac arrest. However, one 21-year-old patient who arrested having received no antidote therapy until 90 min after the attack was successfully resuscitated and was discharged from the hospital after 5 days.

The psychological effects of the sarin release were extensive. Of all the patients seen at the Tokyo hospitals, 74 % had no signs or specific symptoms and were classified as 'worried well'. One month after the event, a survey by St Luke's of more than 600 exposed persons showed that 60 % had symptoms consistent with post-traumatic stress disorder.

Although the number of fatalities was relatively low, the medical impact of the attack was considerable. A recent analysis of the casualties by the physicians involved in their care and after the revelations of court proceedings against Aum Shinrikyo showed that there was a considerable variation in the reported number of casualties by the different emergency services. A report published by the Fire Department cited a total of 5493 persons who were treated in 267 medical institutions in Tokyo, including 14 emergency medical departments and 67 hospitals. However, another report said that a total of 6185 casualties were treated at 294 medical institutions.

The Tokyo incident remains the only large-scale single nerve agent release with multiple casualties seen in a civil setting where detailed clinical analysis has been possible.

Key lessons learned were as follows:

1. The Matsumoto and Tokyo sarin incidents were the first examples of terrorist attacks in a civil setting using a military nerve agent. The sarin used had been synthesised in a secret laboratory and proved that such syntheses were within the capability of terrorist organisations.

2. The effects of the nerve agent release were variable, and the ratio of dead-to-wounded was low. The cause of death was respiratory failure.
3. Medical responders themselves became victims of secondary contamination from the original attack.

Key medical perceptions by attending physicians following the incident were as follows:

1. Severely affected patients needed intermittent positive pressure ventilation (IPPV) due to convulsions and respiratory arrest.
2. Moderately affected patients presented with respiratory distress and fasciculations (there was difficulty in distinguishing between fasciculations and convulsions).
3. Mildly affected patients had only eye symptoms.

Other key medical lessons from the Tokyo incident were as follows:

1. There is a need for emergency medical services to expect the unexpected in relation to toxic agent release.
2. Training and protection of emergency medical teams responding to toxic agent releases are essential to prevent secondary casualties.
3. There was considerable confusion in the Tokyo attack about what had been released and in the distribution of casualties. However, the triage system was probably responsible for saving a number of lives among those who were severely affected by sarin.

10.3.6   2002: The Moscow Theatre Incident

On 23 October 2002, more than 950 people in the Dubrovka Theatre, Moscow, were taken hostage by 40–50 heavily armed Chechen terrorists, who, during a performance of a play, entered the building and threatened to blow it up. About 58 hostages were released on grounds of age and medical conditions. The siege ended on October 26, after an attack by Russian special alpha forces wearing filtration respirators. An inhalational 'knockdown' agent was introduced through the air conditioning system. The agent was supposed to render both the captors and captives unconscious but in the event at least 129 hostages and 42 terrorists died following inhalation of the agent. One hundred and fifty survivors required prolonged hospitalisation. Twelve days after the attack, 67 hostages and 12 rescuers remained hospitalised, with 5 in a critical condition. It is likely that just more than 900 persons were present in the theatre when it was recaptured, and the actual number of deaths from the effects of the gas may have been greater than 200 with scores more left seriously ill in hospital.

An early statement by the Russian authorities said that a 'calmative' agent had been used during the attack to end the siege. Four days after the ending of the siege, the Russian Minister of Health explained that the intention of the special forces attack had been to use a 'calmative' agent that was not essentially toxic to eliminate resistance from the terrorists and render them incapable of detonating the explosives with which they were threatening the hostages. Later, the authorities explained that the agent used was a fentanyl incapacitating agent (see Chap. 3), and it was not essentially harmful, unlike conventional agents of chemical warfare. The exact identity of the fentanyl compound was never revealed.

The nature of this attack and the fatalities caused led to much speculation in the press about what compound might have been used and why the attack had gone wrong, given the loss of life among the hostages. A number of publications considered the attack from a toxicological standpoint and there was correspondence from anaesthesiologists which challenged the explanation of events on the basis of experience from standard anaesthetic practice (where fentanyls are used on an everyday basis).

Some information about the medical aspects of the ending of the siege was available from press and eyewitness accounts. Following the siege, patients admitted to the hospitals were placed under armed guard with very limited access, apparently for fear that some of them might have been terrorists. There appeared to have been no published medical articles about the management of the hospitalised cases in contrast with the large number of peer-reviewed articles, which appeared following the Tokyo sarin incident in 1995. Casualties from the gas release were initially denied by the authorities for 3 days. Despite this, it is possible to put together a sequence of events which may be summarised as follows:

1. The gas was said to have been released at 0500 h, and the first victims removed at 0700 h. However, other reports indicate that the gas may have been released earlier but the concentration had to be increased since it was not having any effect. One Russian website said that special forces began pumping the gas into the building at about 0430 h on October 23. Other sources say that gas pumping began as early as 0100 h and there was speculation that the dose rate may have been increased after failing to act quickly enough early on. One report noted that the gas took effect within 30 min of first being noticed and was visible as a 'smoke' from the air conditioning system. Chechen hostage takers on stage were less affected than people in the stalls and started firing. The battle continued for one-and-a-half hours.
2. The faces of the victims were waxy, white and drawn, eyes open and blank and some of the victims choked in their vomitus.
3. The initial assault was made by special forces wearing special protective equipment and respirators after the gas release. Later, unprotected Ministry of the Interior Forces entered the auditorium but were overcome by gas and started to vomit.
4. Few ambulances were standing by to receive casualties, and buses were commandeered to remove them. This may indicate that the response to the gas took the security forces by surprise.

5. Many accounts note the respiratory failure and vomiting as general signs following the release of the gas. Most of the fatalities in the theatre were apparently caused by respiratory failure. Examination of news footage after the release of the agent shows that there was little attempt at providing airway and ventilatory support. One news story stated that military advice to stockpile naloxone (a widely used opioid antidote) had been given to civil hospitals some days before the attack, but there were other reports of doctors trying a number of antidotes to try to revive casualties who were unconscious and in respiratory failure.

The key medical lessons from this incident are the following:

1. Casualties with toxic trauma may present without any prior knowledge about the nature of the causative agent.
2. The early provision of airway and respiratory life support would have reduced the fatality rate considerably. Video footage from the incident shows casualties being loaded into buses without even a basic attempt at secure left lateral positioning and opening the airway (Fig. 10.2).

10.3.7 1984: Accidental Release of Methyl Isocyanate, Bhopal, India

On the evening of 2 December 1984, there was an explosive leak from a chemical plant in the city of Bhopal in central India (population 900,000). About 27 t of the TIC methyl isocyanate was released and formed a dense cloud over the city which was slow moving. The cloud covered an area of about 40 km^2 of the surrounding city which was densely populated by poor and largely uneducated people. Approximately, 500,000 persons were exposed, and there were estimated 3500–15,000 deaths over a short term.

Fig. 10.2 Casualties with respiratory failure loaded into a bus following the Moscow Theatre siege. No attempt appears to have been made to provide respiratory support nor even to put the casualties into the recovery position (*Source* Wikimedia Commons)

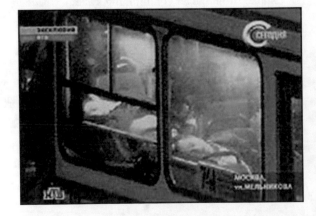

Affected casualties suffered from initial acute airway irritation and inflammatory changes and later from toxic pulmonary oedema. Although the cloud may have contained contaminants and by-products including hydrogen cyanide and oxides of nitrogen, there is little doubt that the main effects were caused by methyl isocyanate which is a known pulmonary oedemagen. Following the release, about 400,000 persons fled the city in a totally uncontrolled evacuation. The evacuation of those who were actually exposed was compounded by a panic evacuation of residents who lived more than 10 km from the release site.

The local medical system which contained 300 doctors and 1800 beds was totally overwhelmed. There was little or no equipment to manage airway and ventilation, and most of the deaths that occurred were from respiratory failure.

Bhopal was the first large-scale release of TIC in a civil setting and provided a number of important lessons in the management of mass casualties following a toxic agent release. These were as follows:

1. A large-scale chemical plant was sited in close proximity to a residential area. Government attempts to persuade the population to move away were resisted by residents who did not wish to move away from a secure source of work.
2. There had been no emergency service planning for a chemical event, nor any emergency medical services special training. Equally there was no chemical hospital disaster plan.
3. There was no community awareness of alarm signals, nor any evacuation plan.
4. The panic evacuation increased the toxic dose of minimum inhibitory concentration (MIC) to the casualties by increasing their respiratory minute volume while running. There was effectively an enhancement of the Haber effect.
5. Some families sheltered inside their home instead of running away and survived.
6. Medical teams were unaware of what had been released from the plant and the potential effects, and there was inadequate medical knowledge about the possible danger or training to respond.
7. The medical response was hampered by inadequate stocks of equipment to provide respiratory support.
8. In terms of its unexpected nature, the Bhopal release was an equivalent of the first chlorine attack in World War I with equally devastating results.
9. The incident acted as an alarm signal around the world for the need for training, equipment and planning to deal with a mass toxic release.
10. The incident had both acute and long-term consequences. The company operating the plant, Union Carbide, established a hospital in Bhopal to care for the victims which is still treating long-term respiratory disease almost 30 years after the event.

10.3.8 Chemical Attacks on Civilians During the Syrian Civil War

At the time of writing, the Syrian Civil War, with its increasing complexity, has raged for over 4 years since 2012. During this time, many thousands of civilians have been killed and wounded as a result of the fighting, much of it in densely populated urban areas. There have been several reports of the use of chemical warfare agents during the fighting but none was investigated until the much-reported attack which occurred during the night of 21 August 2013 in the area of Ghouta (Fig. 10.3). The exact details of this are still sketchy but are the subject of a United Nations report. What this report has made clear, is that a chemical agent, probably sarin, was released during an urban engagement and caused probably more than a thousand dead and wounded. Video footage taken at casualty reception points showed a confused picture of walking and non-walking injured with attempts made at respiratory support. Detailed information was, however, lacking, and there have been accusations and counter accusations of disinformation by both sides of the conflict. Pictures of fatalities have been said to have been manipulated or even posed (as was possibly the case in the reporting from Hallabja), and there have been queries about why the use of a chemical weapon in an urban conflict taking place close to where UN weapon inspectors were based would have been expected to go undetected.

The facts about the attack, as far as they could be established (based upon UN statements, following a report by weapons inspections teams, and from a synopsis of information from the BBC) may be summarised as follows:

1. The first-reported use of chemical warfare agents during an attack came at 0245 h on the morning of 21 August in Ein Tarma, about 6 km from the centre of Damascus and again at 0247 h in adjoining Zamalka. Reports from human rights organisations, based upon evidence from activists in Syria, said that at least eight rockets fell on four sites. These rockets were later identified as being Soviet era M 14 surface to surface 140-mm rockets capable of carrying a 2 kg chemical payload. The remains of other larger 320-mm rockets were later found in the target areas by UN weapons inspectors.

Fig. 10.3 Casualties following the chemical attack in Ghouta, Damascus in 2014. (*Source* Wikimedia Commons https://www.youtube.com/watch?v=yp_Ju6742Z0)

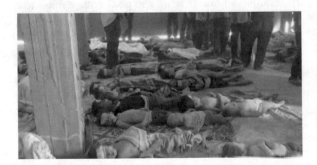

2. Eyewitnesses interviewed later by the UN investigating team reported that large numbers of people were affected a short time after the accident with symptoms that included dyspnoea, disorientation, blurred vision, nausea, vomiting and general weakness. Later, many of those exposed lost consciousness and collapsed.

3. Within hours of the attack, dozens of video clips were uploaded on to the Internet showing neatly laid out shrouded apparent fatalities on the floors of clinics and mosques. The videos also showed victims who were reported to be suffering from the symptoms listed above. Some were seen to be in apparent respiratory distress and were being given free-flow oxygen by face mask, but there were no apparent cases receiving intermittent positive pressure ventilation. Clips shown by television channels were not of sufficient length or detail to be able to present a clear clinical picture of an organophosphate toxidrome. However, from the outset of the reporting, the assumption was made that the cause of the chemical casualties was sarin.

4. A statement by the UN Secretary General Ban Ki-moon on 16 September, after an investigation of the attack sites and survivors by a UN inspection team said that there was 'clear and convincing evidence that sarin was used during the attack and that many hundreds of people were killed'. The inspection team said they had found samples of sarin on the remains of rockets found on the area and that 85 % of blood samples tested from 50 survivors interviewed showed positive for sarin. Details of what tests were carried out were not provided, but red-cell acetylcholinesterase levels, the best indicator of whether exposure to an anticholinesterase has taken place, have not been published at the time of writing.

5. There followed many allegations and counter allegations of who carried out the attack and what the actual death toll was. This was initially reported by the main Syrian Opposition Alliance as being 300, but this had changed to 1,300 by the end of 21 August. A US government assessment put the toll at 1,429 while other human rights organisations (using information from eyewitnesses in Syria) and French intelligence (based upon an analysis of the many online videos placed the death toll at between 280 and 500).

6. Following the attack, Syria acceded in October 2013 to the 1992 chemical weapons convention, the government declared formally the existence of its chemical weapons stocks (which had been suspected for many decades) and steps were started at the end of 2013 to secure their destruction.

Medical lessons from the chemical attacks in Syria The August 2013 chemical attack in Damascus provided a dramatic reminder of the constant threat of sudden and unexpected exposure to toxic chemical agents and the medical consequences of the toxic trauma they produced.

Much uncertainty still surrounds the medical aspects of the incident. Although the UN report concludes beyond doubt that sarin was used in the attack, the video pictures presented by the media do not provide a totally conclusive picture of an organophosphate toxidrome. What is clear, however, is that a chemical attack took place, and the UN concludes that sarin was used. Given the extreme sensitivity of the use of chemical weapons in modern society and the propaganda leverage they provide, it is possible that some of the pictures shown following the Damascus attack were staged to provide additional impact to what had been a genuine chemical attack with a large number of fatalities. The neat rows of shrouded fatalities contrast strangely with the chaotic scenes of casualty reception facilities, although the videos were posted at the same time. This is a reminder of the same effect the pictures sent from Hallabja had in 1988 where some of the casualties had possibly been repositioned post-mortem for added dramatic effects.

Despite the continuing debate and lack of peer-reviewed medical evidence that surrounds the Damascus incident, what is known overall provides important and relevant lessons for those faced with the unexpected management of toxic trauma as a result of the release of a chemical warfare agent or toxic industrial chemical. These illustrate many of the points presented earlier in this book and may be summarised as follows:

1. The attack was unexpected and unpredicted. It took place during the night in the middle of fierce fighting which produced a large number of conventional trauma casualties which had stretched the already overloaded emergency medical facilities.
2. Large numbers of casualties arrived at emergency facilities at the same time, either walking or carried by relatives. The video footage taken apparently on mobile phones showed an uncontrolled system of patient management which did not show any apparent triage attempts. Protective equipment for medical staff was not present, but there were some attempts at decontamination by simple washing with water.
3. Casualties presented or were carried to emergency reception points without any evidence of physical trauma and apparently suffering from severe respiratory distress or total failure. The video footage did not show clear signs of acute respiratory failure in many of the cases although this must be assumed to be the cause of death in the cases of exposure to sarin.
4. Despite reports of aspects of a muscarinic toxidrome, there was no clear initial toxic cause of the mass presentation of casualties. Sarin was mentioned as a probable cause early in the reporting, possibly since this nerve agent is high in media and public awareness since the Matsumoto and Tokyo attacks in 1994–1995. The presence of sarin at the attack site and in survivors was confirmed by the UN investigating teams later. However, the possibility that other chemical agents could have been used at the same time as sarin in the attack (to disguise a clear toxidrome) does not appear to have been considered openly. The use of an incapacitating agent could have led to many of the signs and symptoms seen on the video footage.
5. The scenes in the casualty reception areas appeared chaotic with little or no visible attempts at triage, and decontamination measures were limited to simple washing with water in some of the footage. Personal protective equipment for

the medical responders was apparently lacking. There were reports of evidence of secondary effects on the medical responders and even of fatalities.

6. According to interviewed emergency medical physicians, the main support provided to the casualties was in the form of atropine, of which there was an immediate shortage. There appeared to be little awareness that atropine would not affect the neuromuscular paralysis which was the cause of the observed life-threatening respiratory failure. Although some casualties were seen to be being given free-flow oxygen by a face mask, there were no obvious coordinated attempts at establishing the airway and providing intermittent positive pressure ventilation.

7. The incident provides many lessons which reinforce the need for management of both the incident and the casualties, particularly, the need for organisation of the reception and the prevention of secondary casualties among the emergency medical response teams. Importantly, it illustrates the confusion and panic that surrounds any possibility of the use of a chemical agents and the need for careful application of appropriate measures for the management of casualties. This is particularly true in the provision of airway and ventilation management which was highlighted in Chap. 7.

The 2013 Damascus incident led to the destruction of Syrian chemical munitions by the UN and the Organisation for the Prohibition of Chemical Weapons (OPCW) teams. However, the incident highlights the need for constant awareness by emergency medical responders of the possibility of the deliberate release of toxic chemical agents in a civil setting and of the need to be able to respond in a way that parallels management of conventional trauma. With the possible dissemination of chemical weapons around the world, following the end of the Cold War and the availability of toxic industrial chemicals that could be used by terrorist organisations to create disruption and panic in the general public, emergency medical responders must continue to expect the unexpected. Despite the OPCW action chemical attacks on civilians have continued during the Syrian Civil War. Information from the UN, OPCW and other sources indicates that between 2012 and early 2016, there have been at least 60 confirmed or suspected attacks. These have involved the use of nerve and sulphur mustard agents and chlorine. Over 14,000 persons are thought to have suffered toxic trauma with 1500 fatalities. Not all the attacks can be confirmed, but the figures show that the use of CW agents has continued to increase, notably during 2015 before the Spring 2016 ceasefire at the time of writing. A development in this escalation has been the reported use of chemical weapons by ISIL against Kurdish fighters. This has raised the concern that chemical agents may become part of the ISIL's terrorist activities elsewhere in the world.

10.4   Responding to the Hazards of Toxic Trauma

The examples of chemical incidents above provide important lessons for emergency medical responders who may have to deal with the management of mass casualties following the release of a toxic chemical agent. These should be integrated into a planned approach for an effective response to such an incident.

There are two main stages in the management of toxic trauma, pre-hospital and hospital. Life-saving and other treatment must be provided seamlessly in both settings. In particular, provision of early treatment at the site of release of the toxic agent is of vital importance where the actions are of short latency and there is risk of death from respiratory failure.

Although the division of care between pre-hospital and hospital care is convenient for organisational purposes, it should be remembered that planning systems for hazardous materials (HAZMAT) may not always function and that contaminated patients may arrive in large numbers directly at hospital. The operation of emergency services plans for toxic releases may be confounded by the fear that underlies the public conception of chemical agents being 'weapons of mass destruction'.

10.4.1   Planning and Preparation

The following points are important in planning a safe and effective treatment response to toxic trauma:

1. The overall approach to management must be based on knowledge of the incident and the properties of the agents causing toxic trauma. In particular, the potential hazards to medical responders from secondary contamination must be borne in mind.
2. A working knowledge of the pathophysiology of the effects of toxic agents on body systems is essential.
3. Casualties with toxic trauma may include adults and extremes of age. The young and old are vulnerable subpopulations who require modification of antidote dosage.
4. Rational treatment of toxic trauma must include both life support and antidote measures.
5. Depending on the circumstances of the release, there may be mass casualties presenting at the hospital emergency department which could rapidly overrun the available resources. Planning for toxic trauma management is therefore an essential part of the hospital disaster planning and should integrate the management of both physical and toxic trauma. This is particularly important in the modern urban setting where the possibility of terrorist attack is high.
6. It is important to remember that the 'incident site' can potentially spread to the hospital itself and can place emergency response and other staff in potential

danger, themselves becoming secondary casualties as was the case at St. Luke's Hospital in Tokyo. Although the secondary effects may be relatively mild, they can cause incapacitation and loss of medical effectiveness.

7. Hospital emergency departments must consider themselves part of the overall response which starts with the HAZMAT organisational, rescue primary medical care and decontamination on site. Contact must be established and maintained with the on-site emergency teams and particularly with the ambulance services who are involved in the evacuation to ensure that patients are properly triaged and distributed to the receiving hospitals available.

8. Essential stocks of emergency life-support equipment must be maintained at hospitals designated to receive casualties following a chemical agent release. These must be supplemented by a decontamination facility and supplies of personal protective equipment. As an absolute basis, it is essential that all personnel who may be working in any area receiving hitherto undiagnosed contaminated casualties should have immediate access to a filtration respirator and gloves. Training in the use of protective equipment and performing essential emergency medical tasks while wearing it is of great importance.

9. Previous mass chemical incidents have shown that because of a perception in the general public that toxic chemical agents are 'weapons of mass destruction' against which there is no response the flow of genuine patients with toxic trauma is compounded by a large influx of worried well who may compromise treatment for those in high triage classes. Preparation must therefore be made to receive such persons in the hospital away from the main casualty stream. Counselling and reassurance will be required for potentially large numbers.

10. Because of the fear among the general public about chemical agents, it is essential that medical teams take a positive response in their approach to patient management and to emphasise that it is possible to treat toxic trauma effectively and that mass exposure does not mean mass fatalities.

10.5   Conclusions

There are many medical lessons to be learned from the releases of toxic chemical agents in war and peace over the past 100 years. Although the use of chemical agents is controlled by international treaty in warfare, they have been used again recently in the Syrian Civil War, and there is a continuing risk of the use of such agents in a civil setting by terrorist organisations. The risk of exposure following accidental release of toxic industrial chemicals also remains considerable, particularly in poor developing nations.

The management of casualties following toxic agent release must be integrated into hospital disaster plans, and appropriate equipment and training should be provided.

Further Reading (update)

Dunlop JB (2006) The 2002 Dubrovka and 2004 Beslan hostage crises: a critique of Russian counter—terrorism. Ibidem Verlag, Stuttgart

Hill BA (2008) History of the medical management of chemical casualties. In: Tuorinsky SD (ed) Medical aspects of chemical warfare office of the surgeon general, US army. Borden Institute, Washington DC, pp 77–114 (Chap. 3)

Lapierre D, Moro J (2002) Five past midnight in Bhopal. Simon and Schuster, London

Mehta PS, Mehta AS, Mehta SJ, Makhijani AB (1990) Bhopal tragedy's health effects: a review of methyl isocyanate toxicity. JAMA 264:2781

Moles TM, Baker DJ (1999) Clinical analogies for the management of toxic trauma. Resuscitation 42(2):117–124

Okumura T, Nomura T, Suzuki T et al (2007) The dark morning: the experiences and lessons learned from the Tokyo subway sarin attack. In: Marrs TC, Maynard RL, Sidell FR (eds) Chemical warfare agents: toxicology and treatment, 2nd edn. Wiley, Chichester, pp 277–286 (Chap. 13)

Syria Chemical Attack: What We Know. www.bbc.uk/news/world-middleeast-23927399. Accessed 14 Oct. 2013

United Nations Mission to Investigate Allegations of the Use of Chemical Weapons in the Syrian Arab Republic: Report on the Alleged Use of Chemical Weapons in the Ghouta Area of Damascus on 21 August 2013. www.un.org/disarmament/content/slideshow/Secretary_General_Report_CW_Investigations.pdf. Accessed 14 Oct. 2013

Urbanetti J, Newmark J (2010) Clinical aspects of large scale chemical events. In: Koenig KL, Schultz CH (eds) Disaster medicine: comprehensive principles and practices. Cambridge University Press, New York

Chapter 11
Toxins

Abstract Toxins are chemical substances which are produced in nature by living organisms ranging from bacteria to venomous reptiles and arachnoids. The extreme toxicity of some toxins has led to interest in their possible use in warfare. However, they are classified by international convention with biological warfare agents and not as chemical agents. As with chemical warfare agents and toxic industrial chemicals, toxins act on a number of somatic systems giving rise to signs and symptoms that resemble chemical agents. However, their molecular size makes them immunologically active, and toxoids exist for the treatment of the effects of many toxins, unlike chemical warfare agents. This chapter considers the classification and actions of toxins which may cause toxic trauma through deliberate release warfare or from terrorist action. The management of the actions of toxins from natural causes such as snakebite is outside the scope of the discussion presented here but is the subject of many specialised toxicological texts

11.1 Introduction

The discussion in this book has concerned toxic hazards classified as agents of chemical warfare or toxic industrial chemicals. The production, weaponisation and stockpiling and use of chemical weapons are banned by international convention. Toxins are by nature biological in origin and are not covered by the same conventions as chemical agents. They are, by definition, chemical substances which are produced from living organisms, ranging from pathogenic bacteria to venomous arachnoids and reptiles. Toxins produce toxic trauma through a variety of mechanisms affecting several body systems. They have been the target of a great deal of research over the past 50 years because of their potential as chemical agents which would be outside the remit of the chemical weapons conventions. The deliberate release of pathogens as agents of biological warfare is outside the remit of this book (although an introduction to the subject is provided in Chap. 12), as is the biochemical actions of pathogens in their natural setting. However, since toxins which

© Springer International Publishing Switzerland 2016

D.J. Baker, *Toxic Trauma*, DOI 10.1007/978-3-319-40916-0_11

are produced by self-replicating organisms have toxic trauma actions on the systems of the body, the object of this chapter was to provide a basic introduction to toxins for the non-specialist reader. The discussion will concern the classification and actions of toxins which may cause toxic trauma through deliberate release warfare or from terrorist action, together with essentials of management. The management of the actions of toxins from natural causes such as snake or spider bites is outside the scope of the discussion presented but is covered by several specialised toxicological texts (see suggestions for further reading).

11.2   Definitions and the Natural History of Toxins

A toxin is any chemical toxic substance that can be produced by a biological organism including animal, plant or microbe. Some toxins can also be produced by molecular biological techniques or by chemical synthesis. Although toxins are produced by self-replicating biological systems they are themselves essentially chemical in nature and do not replicate. Toxins are the means by which one organism can cause harm to another. Examples are widespread in nature and range from envenomation following snake or insect bites to the production of toxins by bacteria following an infection. Familiar examples of bacterial infection causing toxin-induced toxic trauma include plague, cholera and anthrax. Clostridium botulinum produces botulinum toxin which causes a severe form of food poisoning from eating poorly canned food. It should be noted that although bacteria cause damage in the body via toxins, this is not the case with viruses which interfere directly with the internal metabolism of the body cells.

11.3   Classification

Toxins may be classified in a number of ways according to whether they are of high or low molecular weight (MW) and whether or not they are proteins. Low MW toxins typically have a weight of 1000 Daltons or about that of 10 amino acids. Toxins classed as protein toxins are generally composed of more than ten amino acids. Classification in terms of molecular weight is useful since toxicity is broadly a function of increasing size. Toxins are also commonly classified in terms of their biological origin such as marine toxins or relating to the body system on which they act, such as neurotoxins or enterotoxins.

11.4   Actions of Toxins in Humans

Toxins harm the human organism by being produced in situ by bacterial infection, by ingestion (food poisoning) or by injection (from poisonous snakes and insects). Compared with chemical agents, toxins are not usually dermally active and are non-volatile. Exceptions to this rule are trichothecenes and cyanotoxin which cause toxicity through the dermal route. During the Vietnam War, T2 trichothecene toxin (Yellow Rain) was thought to be the cause of an outbreak of skin and systemic disease among the Hmong tribesmen in Cambodia. Toxins act almost on all the systems of the body, but their mechanisms of action do not correlate with their classification, molecular weight and biological origins.

11.5   Use of Toxins as Research Tools

Because many toxins have highly specific actions at receptors and at ion channels they have found much use as laboratory research tools to elucidate basic biological mechanisms. Black widow spider venom and alpha-bungarotoxin from the cobra are classic examples which block the acetylcholine (ACh) receptor at the neuro-muscular junction.

   These and other neurotoxins such as tetrodotoxin (which blocks the transmission of signals along motor nerves by interference with the passage of sodium ions through the membrane surrounding the nerve) have been used for many years in neurophysiological research.

11.6   Toxins and Toxoids

For many years, toxoids, which are immunologically active but non-toxic derivatives of toxins, have been used as in the prophylaxis and treatment of bacterial toxin-related diseases. These include notably diphtheria and botulism. Toxins must be produced as an essential precursor to the production of antitoxins and thus potential stocks of toxins exist from this route, which are produced in large-scale fermentation tanks. The existence of such stocks, which were outside the existing Chemical Weapons Convention, was the initial source of suspicion that toxins were being developed for use as toxic agents by the Soviet Union during the Cold War in the 1980s.

11.7   Toxicity

Toxins are among the most poisonous substances known to humans. However, detailed information about their toxicity in humans is often not available, and extrapolations have to be made from studies in experimental animals.

   Toxicity is usually expressed as an LD_{50} value and is typically expressed in mg of material per kg of subject-body weight. The LD_{50} values are usually derived from populations of mice and then extrapolated in humans to calculate the toxic dose levels. A toxin with an LD_{50} of <0.025 µg/kg is regarded as being among the most highly toxic, an example being botulinum toxin (BoTx) with an LD_{50} of 0.001 µg/kg.

Although toxins usually act via ingestion (e.g. food poisoning) or injection (envenomation) recent research indicates that they can act by inhalation in the case of a deliberate military or terrorist release. In this situation, the toxicity value should be assessed by a LCt_{50} value as for inhaled chemical agents. However, for the most part, data are lacking.

11.8 Comparison of Toxins with Chemical Warfare Agents

Toxins are placed midway between a spectrum of hazards that exists between chemical and biological warfare agents. Unlike biological agents, they are not self-replicating although they are classed with biological warfare agents by international convention. Table 11.1 shows a comparison of toxins with conventional chemical agents.

11.9 Toxin Release: Factors Affecting Practical Toxicity

Toxicity, difficulty of production and delivery systems are limiting factors when considering toxins as mass casualty agents. Toxicity alone is not always the determining factor of hazard.

In their natural mode of transmission to humans, the environmental hazards of toxins are well documented. Insect and snake bites are good examples.

Table 11.1 Comparison of toxins with chemical agents

Toxins	Chemical warfare agents
Natural origins. Complex chemical structure	Man made. Usually low molecular weight and simple chemical structure
Synthesis difficult in most cases by large-scale production possible by fermentation techniques	Large-scale industrial production possible in all cases
Non-volatile but can be aerosolised	Many are volatile and active through the inhaled route
Legitimate medical use in some cases (e.g. BoTx)	No legitimate medical use. Industrial feedstocks as TIC in some cases
Odourless and tasteless	Most agents have detectable odour and taste
Diverse toxic effects on body systems. Immunologically active	Simpler toxic effects on respiratory, nervous skin and mucous membranes. Generally immunologically inactive
Aerosol delivery through the inhaled route	Gas, vapour aerosol and mist delivery via the inhaled route

Hazards from deliberate airborne release of toxins for harmful purposes are not so well understood. During the Cold War, there was considerable research into the possible use of toxins spread by aerosol and introduced into the body through the lungs. This mode of transmission is not usual in nature, and many of the details of toxicity of toxins encountered in this way remain unpublished. However, some work published openly confirms that a toxin such as botulinum, normally transmitted by the oral route as a food poison, is active in this way.

The hazards presented by toxins dispersed by an atypical aerosol route include stability and the ability to remain in an aerosol (particles greater than 15–20 microns fall out of the aerosol). The retention of particles within the terminal bronchioles and alveoli of the lung is also a factor. They achieve entry in this way (particles must be less than two microns in diameter).

11.10   Hazards and Threats: The Deliberate Release of Toxins for Harmful Purposes

The Australia Group has compiled an open list (Box 11.1) of toxins that have the potential for misuse. This list contains toxins from marine, bacterial, plant and fungal origin.

Box 11.1 Toxins from marine, bacterial, plant and fungal origins that have potential for misuse by deliberate release
Botulinum toxin (BoTx)
Clostridium perfringens toxins
Conotoxin
Ricin
Saxitoxin
Shiga toxin
Staphylococcus enterotoxin B (SEB)
Tetrodotoxin
Verotoxin
Microcystin
Aflatoxin (AFB1)
Abrin
Cholera toxin
Diacetoxyscirpenol (DAS)
T-2 toxin
HT-2 toxin
Modeccin toxin
Volkensin toxin
Viscumin toxin

Table 11.2 Laboratory toxicity values of the toxins in Box 11.1

Botulinum	0.001 µg/kg
Shiga toxin	0.002 µg/kg
Verotoxin	0.2 µg/kg
Volkensin	1.38 µg/kg
Ricin	2 µg/kg
Tetrodotoxin	8 µg/kg
Saxitoxin	8 µg/kg
Conotoxin	12 µg/kg
Abrin	20 µg/kg
SEB	27 µg/kg
CPT	39 µg/kg
Viscumin	80 µg/kg
Microcystin-LR	127 µg/kg
Cholera toxin	260 µg/kg
Modeccin	2.3 mg/kg
T-2	5.2 mg/kg
HT-2	6.5 mg/kg
DAS	7.8 mg/kg
AFB$_1$	9.5 mg/kg

Table 11.2 gives laboratory toxicity values for this group based upon intraperitoneal injection in mice. This highlights the wide range of toxicity derived in this manner.

11.11 Neurotoxin Hazards

The toxin BoTx, produced by the anaerobe *Clostridium botulinum,* has the reputation of being the most toxic substance by weight known to humans, being at least 5000 times more toxic than sarin. Botulism is a disease of both humans and animals. Seven different functionally related neurotoxins are produced by various strains (A–G). Botulism is essentially an intoxication, brought on by ingestion of the toxin produced by clostridial infection of food, usually incorrectly canned meats. Primary botulism, a direct infection, is rare and only affects infants in the human species. Botulinum intoxication can, however, be treated, and this modifies the toxicity considerably. It is estimated that less than 10 % of natural cases receiving ventilatory and antitoxin support are fatal.

BoTx acts at the nerve terminal of cholinergic synapses and blocks the release of ACh (see Chap. 6), after being taken up into the vesicles and translocated to the cytoplasm where the toxin catalyses proteolysis of components involved in the calcium-mediated exocytosis of ACh. The inhibition is permanent, and recovery occurs only after the creation of new terminal boutons. The toxin thus blocks neurotransmission, parasympathetic synapses and peripheral ganglia. Conventionally after ingestion of the toxin (the usual route), the parasympathetic action produces a dry mouth, followed by signs of a progressive bulbar palsy (dysarthria, dysphasia and dysphagia) and ocular signs (diplopia and ptosis). Following this, there is a progressive symmetrical descending muscular weakness leading to respiratory failure requiring prolonged ventilatory support. NM testing shows a classical presynaptic decremental pattern to repeated stimuli with post-tetanic facilitation. Single-fibre electromyography (see Box 9.1) will detect the neuromuscular changes before conventional nerve stimulation; there is increased jitter and blocking which is reduced by increasing the nerve firing rate. The pattern of signs and symptoms following a deliberate mass inhalation release is not known, but BoTx must be considered along with the nerve agents in any cases presenting with sudden cholinergic features.

Saxitoxin (STX) and tetrodotoxin (TTX) are very potent neurotoxins. Unlike BoTx, they act by blocking the sodium ion channels along the nerve that are essential for nerve impulse transmission, leading to sensory and motor nerve dysfunction.

Both STX and TTX are difficult to cultivate and purify from natural sources and cannot be synthesised chemically. However, they may be a hazard through contamination of food sources such as sea food grown in contaminated water, which could lead to bioaccumulation of large quantities of STX. It is also a heat-stable toxin which would mean that contaminated food could not be easily decontaminated.

11.12   DNA Toxin Hazards

The toxins ricin and abrin cause widespread damage to DNA in the body leading to multiple organ failure. Until recently, it was thought that they could only be introduced into the body by an injection, but there are indications that they could be active by inhalation of an aerosol. Ricin can be extracted from castor oil plants and there have been reported attempts to do this by terrorist cells. Ricin is highly toxic and was used in the assassination of the Bulgarian diplomat Georgi Markov in London in 1978. At present, there is no specific antidote for toxic trauma caused by ricin.

11.13   Applied Toxicity of Toxins

In order to assess dangers posed from the storage and use of toxins factors other than conventional expressions of laboratory, toxicity must be taken into account. These have been indicated above and include stability, ability to be aerosolised, pathophysiological actions and effectiveness of prophylactic and therapeutic measures.

On this basis, hazards presented by the synthesis and storage of toxins can be graded for purposes of security where there is a concern that deliberate release may be an objective. In this way, toxins in an urban society may be classified as high, medium and low risk in terms of the overall hazard presented, assuming that medical countermeasures are available.

11.13.1 High-Risk Toxins

On the basis of the considerations above, the greatest hazards are posed by DNA toxins such as ricin and abrin. These can be produced easily and are relatively stable. They attack multiple organ systems in the body, and there are no specific therapeutic measures other than intensive care support. Available clinical data from accidental and deliberate poisonings support this view.

Ricin is most toxic when inhaled and is therefore a potential aerosol threat. However, large quantities would be needed to cause toxicity. Ricin is much less lethal when ingested, suggesting poor absorption. The toxicity and lethality of parenteral exposure to ricin are well documented. Abrin which is closely related to ricin in structure is extremely toxic with an LD_{50} dose for humans of 2 μg/kg.

11.13.2 Medium-Risk Toxins

The neurotoxins, including saxitoxin, tetrodotoxin, BoTx and conotoxins, pose a major hazard when considered in terms of laboratory toxicity, ease of production, ease of dissemination and the ability to cause high mortality and morbidity. However, respiratory failure, that is the common fatal pathway, can be treated by artificial ventilation, and other specific therapeutic measures are available.

11.13.3 Low-Risk Toxins

Enterotoxins (which normally cause food poisoning) pose the least risk. Mortality rates with the other toxins mentioned such as aflatoxins and the enterotoxins would not have a high mortality, but the morbidity of the release would be quite high. Such toxins should be regarded as essentially agents of mass morbidity but not of mass fatality.

11.13.4   Stability

The stability of the toxins is also an important factor when judging the applied potency of a toxin. A highly toxic but low MW toxin, outside its normal biological environment, may be highly unstable and would not survive the actual delivery system. Stability is a problem with enterotoxins, with most being denatured at higher temperatures or natural fast degradation in the environment. Most of the toxins or the bacteria from which the toxin is produced are denatured in normal water treatment methods. Staphylococcal enterotoxin B is very stable and heat labile which poses as the main hazard in this category. Botulinum and anthrax toxins are also sufficiently robust to withstand weaponisation and delivery.

11.14   Management of Deliberate Toxin Exposure

Deliberate exposure to toxins is based on their essential chemical nature and therefore management follows the measures described in earlier chapters. Although toxins are highly toxic when viewed solely in terms of laboratory study of toxicity, their effects on humans are considerably modified due to medical countermeasures. These include immunological measures such as active immunisation and the administration of antibody therapy. In addition, the provision of non-specific medical countermeasures such as life support to treat impending respiratory failure in the case of paralysing actions alters the toxicity of many toxins by factors of several thousands in many cases. Thus, intoxication by BoTx, whether naturally acquired through ingestion of the toxin following food poisoning or by inhalation of an aerosol, has a very low mortality if treated with ventilatory life support and antitoxins.

While medical countermeasures are effective against the neurotoxins, they are not so against DNA toxins where multiple somatic systems are involved and there is general organ failure.

Food poisonings from staphylococcal enterotoxin B or from botulism, or tetanism, are relatively familiar situations in some emergency departments around the world. However, exposure to other neurotoxins such as saxitoxin or DNA toxins such as ricin is a rarity. Assessment of the patient presenting with signs and symptoms of toxic trauma and the circumstances of the exposure may give clues to any patient who presents with an unusual illness. Guidelines for the management of any unusual illness have been produced in the UK and are cited in the suggestions for further reading.

11.15   Conclusions

Toxins are widespread in nature being produced by bacterial, animal, plant and marine organisms. They are essentially chemical in nature but are not classed as chemical warfare agents. Toxins may be involved in either natural disease or as a result of deliberate release. They have a wide range of toxicity with neurotoxins such as botulinum toxin being the most toxic substance to man by weight. However, conventional laboratory toxicity data for toxins do not reflect the true hazards of agents dispersed in an atypical way to human population within the reach of emergency care facilities. Practical factors which must be taken into account in estimating the hazards posed by toxins are (1) those related to the physical stability and ability to aerosolise the toxin and (2) the effects of medical countermeasures including immunological techniques and life-support measures. In this respect, the management of the effects of toxins has considerable overlap with that of toxic trauma caused by conventional chemical agents. In particular, life support measures remain an essential first line of response.

Further Reading

Alibek K (2002) Biohazard (Chapter 12). Arrow Books, London, UK
Arnon S, Schechter R, Inglesby T et al (2001) Botulinum toxin as a biological weapon. JAMA 285 (8):1059
Harris R, Paxman J (2002) A higher form of killing: the secret history of chemical and biological warfare. Arrow Books, London, UK
Heptonstall J, Gent N (2006) CBRN incidents: clinical management and health protection. Health Protection Agency, London
Karalliedde L (1995) Animal toxins. Br J Anaesth 74(3):319
The Australia Group (2014). www.australiagroup.net. Accessed 03 May 2016
Waite TD, Baker DJ, Murray VSG (2014) Marine toxins. In: Rutty GN (ed) Essentials of autopsy practice. Chapter 3. Springer, London, UK
Williams P, Willens S, Anderson J et al (2007) Toxins: established and emergent threats. In: Tuorinsky SD (ed) Medical aspects of chemical and biological warfare. Office of the Surgeon General, Borden Institute, Walter Reed Hospital (Chap. 19), Washington DC, pp 613–644

Chapter 12
Chemical, Biological, Radiological and Nuclear Hazards: An Overview and Comparison

Abstract Grouping together chemical, biological, radiological and nuclear agents as 'weapons of mass destruction ' (WMD) has been rather uncritically accepted since the appearance of the CBRN classification more than 30 years ago, replacing the original military nuclear, biological and chemical (NBC) classification. Despite the apparent operational convenience of the CBRN grouping from a military and political standpoint, it remains medically unsatisfactory. In reality, there are very considerable differences between the different classes of agent, and only nuclear weapons should be truly regarded as WMD, given the degree of trauma, both physical and from radiation and material destruction they cause. There is often confusion, particularly among civil emergency responders about the real nature of CBRN injuries and the risks they pose to others. This often leads to a negation of the fact that toxic, biological and radiation trauma are inherently treatable and thus mass injury does not necessarily mean mass fatalities. Earlier chapters in this book have considered toxic trauma caused by exposure to toxic chemical agents. This chapter provides a comparison of chemical with biological agents, and with radiation injury. A detailed discussion of biological agents is outside the scope of this book, but radiation injury is covered in more detail, particularly the essential differences between radioactivity (and accompanying possible contamination) and radiation itself, which may be the result of the deliberate release of a radioactive substance or the explosion of a nuclear device. Although chemical, biological, radiological and nuclear agents produce different types of trauma they can be viewed in terms of their essential properties which have been discussed earlier for chemical agents which are as follows: (1) physical form and how the agent interfaces with the body, (2) persistency—how long the agent remains in the environment, (3) toxicity—how the agent causes trauma to the body and (4) latency—the time taken for physical signs and symptoms to appear.

© Springer International Publishing Switzerland 2016
D.J. Baker, *Toxic Trauma*, DOI 10.1007/978-3-319-40916-0_12

12.1   Introduction: The Origins and History of the CBRN Classification

Since the end of the Second World War it has been customary to class harmful agents causing both toxic and extreme physical trauma together. This began with the grouping of Nuclear, Biological and Chemical (NBC) agents at the beginning of the Cold War. Although these agents cause trauma in different ways they were regarded by the military as being so different from conventional weapons of warfare that a separate approach was required for training and protection. Chemical weapons had already been used extensively in the First World War (Chap. 2) and were used in the Abyssinian campaign in 1936 and probably in the Manchurian War from 1932. However, development of the nerve agents in Germany before and during the Second World War in total secrecy provided a completely new hazard and threat. Equally, biological weapons were developed extensively during that period and were tested and possibly used (Paxman and Harris 2002). The development of the atomic bomb which was used at the end of the war against Japan provided another new form of weapon, one which would kill and injure by both physical and radiation trauma, which can be regarded as a special form of toxic trauma.

In the 1970s, the NBC classification was changed by both military and civil formations to include radioactive substances, separate from those produced by a nuclear explosion. This resulted in the CBRN (chemical, biological, radiological and nuclear) classification still in use today. Why the term 'radiological' was chosen to describe the hazards from substances that are radioactive is not clear. The term in English had always been used to describe the medical speciality of imaging by X-rays. However the term has remained unaltered and by convention will be used in this chapter to mean a radioactive substance.

Chapter 2 described the development of chemical weapons from the industrial revolution through the First and Second World Wars and beyond. The rise of the chemical industries following the industrial revolution was the main driving force for the early development of chemical weapons. Equally, the development of bacteriology and virology during the late nineteenth and twentieth centuries laid the foundations for the deliberate release of pathogens against both combatants and civil populations, as biological warfare. Biological warfare (BW) developed later than CW but the risks were realised during and after the First World War and thus BW was also included in the protocols of the 1925 Geneva Convention.

By the 1930s, during the Manchurian War between Japan and China (which some historians regard as the real beginning of World War 2) BW started in its modern format with dispersal of pathogens by air, ground and water contamination. However, the concept of BW was not new, having been used in mediaeval times when corpses infected with plague had been fired over siege walls to infect the enclosed civil population. There was a possible use of incapacitating BW agents against horses during WW1. During WW2 there was a substantial effort to weaponise anthrax by the British who contaminated Gruinard Island in Scotland as part of tests. In Japan, there was an extensive BW development programme by a research station known as unit 731. At the end of WW2, the capture and debriefing by the United States of the principle workers led by Colonel Tojiro Ishii started a BW arms race which lasted throughout the whole of the Cold War, with extensive research conducted by the Soviet Union until its disintegration after the fall of the Berlin Wall (Alibek 2000).

After the industrial revolution and the development of the sciences of bacteriology and virology the third driving force behind the development of CBRN agents was the discovery of nuclear fission in the 1920s and 1930s. With the development of nuclear weapons there was a seismic shift in warfare with the production of a weapon that could cause intense physical damage from an explosive shock wave together with short- and long-term radiation trauma from both direct irradiation from the nuclear explosion and also from later contamination by radioactive isotopes (radioactive fallout).

By 1945, therefore, military planning had to encompass not only physical trauma as a result of penetrating, blunt and blast injury (conventional weapons), but also new forms such as chemical, biological and radiation trauma. Initially the response to these new hazards was to group them together as NBC weapons since, operationally these hazards require protection and decontamination for continued military effectiveness and survival. Special NBC schools and units were set up by both sides during the Cold War with the production of better protective equipment and decontamination techniques as part of the arms race.

The problem with the NBC classification was that it did not sufficiently emphasise the differences between the pathophysiological consequences of exposure to the different classes of agent, particularly in regard to the latency of the appearance of injury. The 1980s saw a reclassification of NBC to CBRN. This change reflected an increasing awareness that radiation injury could be caused by other means than a nuclear explosion. With the rise of international terrorism there was increasing concern about the dispersal of radioactive isotopes by a conventional explosive device (the so-called 'dirty bomb' or improvised radiological dispersion device, IRDD).

12.1.1   The Scope of This Chapter

The CBRN classification has now been universally but rather uncritically accepted and also the components of the classification are equally regarded as being 'weapons of mass destruction'. The validity of this assumption is discussed later. Despite the apparent operational convenience of the NBC and CBRN classifications by the military and civil emergency services, and the use of the mass destruction concept for political leverage, grouping of trauma caused by the individual chemical, biological, radiological and nuclear weapons remains unsatisfactory from a medical standpoint. There is often confusion, particularly among civil emergency responders about the nature of CBRN injuries and the risks they pose to others. This book has considered toxic trauma caused by exposure to toxic chemical agents. This chapter provides an introduction to biological, radiological and nuclear agents for non-specialist emergency medical responders, together with a comparison of the type of trauma they produce. Definitions of chemical, biological, radiological and nuclear agents are shown in Box 12.1. The actions of biological agents are part of the whole subject of infectious disease. A detailed discussion is beyond the scope of this book but as an introduction agents of biological warfare are considered in relation to other members of the CRBN grouping in terms of key properties they have in common. Radioactivity and the trauma caused by exposure to radiation are often not clearly understood by emergency medical responders in the civil setting. The chapter therefore contains a more detailed discussion of this subject to help fill this gap.

Box 12.1 Definitions of chemical, biological, radiological and nuclear agents

Chemical agent	a chemical substance that is intended for use in military and terrorist operations to kill, seriously injure or otherwise incapacitate man through pathophysiological effects
Biological agent	the deliberate release of a bacterial or viral pathogen with the object of infecting man or animals to cause disability or death through pathophysiological effects
Radiological agent	the deliberate release of a radioactive substance by means other than a nuclear explosion to cause radiation injury or death to man
Nuclear agent	A device which causes a very high-energy explosion by the breakup or fusion of atoms causing a massive blast wave accompanied by the release of high-energy electromagnetic radiation as well as dispersed radioisotopes

---

12.2 'Weapons of Mass Destruction' in Perspective

The term 'weapon of mass destruction' has been increasingly used over the past thirty years by politicians, military and civil emergency responders to describe casualties from any attack by a CBRN agent. However, 'mass destruction' if applied to both loss of life and injury together with physical destruction is only applicable to nuclear weapons. Chemical, biological and radiological agents, although they can render an environment uninhabitable do not *per se* cause physical damage of the type caused by the blast wave of a nuclear explosion. The concept of uninhabitability links all CBRN agents since they can all cause contamination which may last from hours to many thousands of years. Such contamination can be countered by decontamination techniques but at a potential cost to human life. Despite the obvious differences between CBRN agents which will be discussed later, the concept of them being 'weapons of mass destruction' has resonated with the general public as well as by military and administrative bodies. The notion that there is an equal response required for protection and decontamination for all CBRN agents has been well-demonstrated by the often standard response to the release of white powders (following the New York anthrax attacks in 2001) where emergency services approach any such incident wearing the highest level of chemical protection, which is not required for biological or radioactive isotope release.

To date, only chemical agent releases in warfare and civil attacks such as those in Hallabja and in Syria (Chap. 10) and the nuclear attacks on Japan in 1945 have produced detailed casualty figures. As mentioned in Chap. 2, analysis of the WW1 chemical casualties shows that the effects of chemical agent exposure were diminished as protective equipment improved and also that the ratio of dead to wounded was lower than that for conventional weapons. Perhaps the greatest threat from CBRN agents is the psychological response they provoke among the general public, particularly from the release of BW agents. This is often way beyond the real risks involved.

12.3 A Brief Overview of Biological Agents of Warfare and Terrorism

In the CBRN classification, a BW agent is defined as a microorganism or a toxin derived from a living organism that can be used in warfare or, more recently, in civil terrorist attacks with the intent of killing or injuring humans, animals or plants. As we have seen in Chap. 11, toxins are essentially chemical in nature, usually consisting of considerably larger molecules than conventional chemical agents. They are however classed as BW agents by international convention because of their natural rather than synthetic origins. Apart from toxins BW agents include bacteria and viruses which are self-replicating. These include pathogens which are known to cause infection, both individual and epidemic in normal natural settings. In the case of an infection which is caused deliberately, a BW pathogen is chosen by the perpetrator because of its high infectivity and the potentially lethal harm caused to the systems of the body. Bacteria, following entry into the body and self-replication cause trauma as a result of the actions of the toxins they produce which is the final pathway of cellular and finally multiorgan damage. In addition they can attack the immune system of the body reducing the natural defences. Bacteria multiply in the body independently, but viruses must invade the cells and take over their metabolic processes in order to be able to replicate.

A wide range of microorganisms have been considered in the past as potential BW agents. Box 12.2 shows a list of potential recognised threats issued by US Center for Disease Control. A further discussion of these is to be found in the suggestions for further reading at the end of this chapter.

Box 12.2 Potential BW agents

Category A bioterrorism agents

  Anthrax

  Plague

  Tularaemia

  Smallpox

  Ebola and Marburg haemorrhagic fevers

Other potential agents include

  Toxins

   Ricin

   Staphylococcal Endotoxin B (SEB)

   Tricothecene mycotoxins

  Bacteria

   Glanders

   Melloidosis

   Brucellosis

  Viruses

   Venezualan Equine Encephalitis (which affects both horses and humans)

  Othermicroorganisms

   Typhus

   Q fever

12.3.1 Routes of Exposure to BW Agents

Delivery of a BW agent is not easy, and the problems associated are discussed below. However, theoretically, three routes are available: inhalation, oral and dermal. In the setting of military action, the inhalation route is considered to be the most likely risk. Scenarios have been considered for the use of this route by terrorists in confined spaces such as an underground railway system.

Key points:

(1) Inhalational. In this route BW agents are dispersed as an aerosol with a small particl size to allow the agent to be inhaled into the terminal bronchi and alveoli of the lung tissue. Such aerosols are potentially odourless, colourless and poorly visible.

(2) Oral. This is a natural route for the ingestion of toxins such as SEB and botulinum which cause food poisoning. After a BW attack, both food and water may become contaminated providing a secondary harmful pathway after the inhalational route.

(3) Dermal. Intact skin provides an effective barrier against penetration by bacteria and viruses. However, infection can be caused by some bacteria, viruses and toxins entering the body through damaged skin if there is associated physical injury.

12.3.2   Recognising a BW Attack

Although there have been military developments in providing mechanical means of detecting a BW aerosol, in the civil setting, where a terrorist attack is currently the most likely threat detection will depend largely on observation. This parallels the use of the senses in detecting a chemical agent release as discussed in Chap. 5.

It is important for emergency medical responders, faced with a potential BW attack to be aware of the essential features which are different from C, R and N releases. These are listed in Box 12.3. Because the effects of a BW attack are more insidious than those of C, R or N attacks and the release is less obvious, it is essential that emergency responders should maintain a high level of suspicion about possible BW agent release.

Box 12.3 Indications of a possible biological agent attack

An outbreak of a disease that is unusual or that does not occur naturally in a given geographical area

Combinations of diseases in the same patient indicating that multiple BW agents may have been released

Unexplained clusters of patients with the same unusual signs and symptoms

Multiple patients presenting with a common latency period after a possible attack by aerosol

The appearance of clusters of dead animals of multiple species

Data suggesting a massive point source or line source release for non-contagious agents (e.g. anthrax)

For individual patients, the following points may indicate a BW release:

- Any unusual illness causing sudden and unexplained febrile death
- Illness that is unusual for the time of year
- Illness that is unusual for the patient's age group
- Illness that is unexplained by environmental contact (e.g. anthrax with no contact with animals or hides)
- Illness that has unusual clinical signs (e.g. mediastinal widening on chest X-ray in anthrax)
- The unusual progression of an illness (e.g. lack of antibiotic response, the presence of a chicken pox like rash on the extremities indicating smallpox)

The UK Department of Health CBRN Handbook notes:

'Any confirmed case of smallpox, plague, glanders, tularaemia, Venezualan equine encephalitis or viral haemorrhagic fever occurring in the UK should be assumed to be the result of deliberate (BW) release until proved otherwise'

12.3.3   Medical Prophylactic and Treatment Measures Against BW Agents

Unlike CW agents, protection against BW agents is possible by vaccination and therefore stimulation of the body immune system. Antitoxins are also available against toxin attack. These may be compared with the antidotes against CW toxic trauma discussed in Chap. 8). In addition, prophylactic antibiotic treatment is possible as was the case during the 2001 terrorist anthrax attacks in New York where doxycycline was widely used. Treatment of BW exposure is however a specialised medical subject, and in the event of a potential attack guidelines are usually issued by the competent State authorities such as CDC in the USA and Public Health England in the UK

12.3.4   The Importance of Latency in BW Agent Exposure

Long latency of clinical expression of signs and symptoms (the equivalent of a natural incubation period) is characteristic of BW compared with CW agents. It is very important for emergency responders to be aware of this when considering the evolution of a syndrome characteristic of a disease compared with chemically induced toxidromes.

12.4   An Introduction to Radiation Injury

Knowledge of the basic science of radioactivity and radiation is important for the understanding of the injuries produced. There is often confusion among emergency medical responders about the cause and nature of these injuries and how they compare with other agents in the CBRN grouping. This section discusses the fundamentals of radiation injury and the way it is caused.

12.4.1   Ionising Radiation

Ionising radiation has been recognised since the nineteenth century when it was first detected from radioactive substances. The French pioneers in this field, Henri Bequerel and Marie Curie (Box 12.4) have given their names to the measurements of radioactivity described below. Ionising radiation, as its name suggests is the transfer of energy to the cells of the body where it creates ions (charged atoms). These are highly reactive and cause damage to both the metabolism and the DNA of the body cells. In some organs of the body, such as the gut and bone marrow the cells divide rapidly as part of their normal activity. It was recognised early on in the study of radiation that the faster the cell divides the more sensitive it is to ionising radiation. This is known as the Bergonie–Tribondau law after the French scientists who first described it. The various forms of radiation injury and the syndromes they produce are a result of the different sensitivities of tissues. There are two types of ionising radiation:

(1) Electromagnetic (wave)
(2) Particle radiation.

Box 12.4 Becquerel and Curie: two great pioneers in the discovery of radioactivity

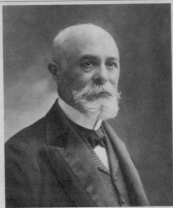

Antoine – Henri Becqueurel

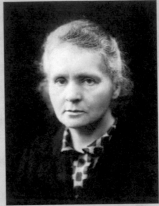

Marie Curie (circa 1920)

Antoine-Henri Becqueurel
Source Wikimedia Commons

Antoine-Henri Becquerel (1852–1908) was born in Paris into a family that produced four generations of scientists, A physicist, he originally studied engineering at the prestigious Ecole Polytechnique in Paris. He later became professor of physics at the Natural History Museum in Paris. Becquerel had always been interested in phosphorescent materials and thought that some of these, such as uranium salts might emit X radiation which had recently been discovered by Roentgen. By accident, he found that a wrapped photographic plate became clouded without exposure to light if placed in contact with a uranium salt. If a piece of metal (a Maltese Cross) was placed between the wrapped plate and the salt its outline was clearly visible. Becquerel had discovered that radiation was coming from the uranium salt. He originally thought that this was due to phosphorescence which had been generated by exposure of the salt to

Marie Curie (circa 1920)
Source Wikimedia Commons

Marie Slowdowska-Curie (1867–1934) was born in Poland but became a French citizen when she married the physicist Pierre Curie. She herself was a distinguished physicist and chemist who was the first woman to win a Nobel prize and the only woman to win one twice. She shared the 1903 prize for physics with Antoine-Henri Becquerel and with her husband and won the 1911 prize for chemistry alone. She worked on the understanding of the science of radioactivity and discovered two new elements, Polonium (named after her country of birth) and Radium. The latter was to provide the earliest form of radiotherapy, a form of treatment which Marie Curie pioneered until her own death from aplastic anaemia as a result of working for many years with unshielded radioactive sources

(continued)

(continued)

sunlight but further experiments lead him
to conclude that the penetrating radiation
reaching the photographic plate was an
intrinsic property of the uranium salt
itself. He had discovered what we now
know to be radioactivity, but he did not
coin that term. Marie Curie had that
distinction

12.4.2   Electromagnetic Radiation

There is a wide range of electromagnetic radiation which is shown in Fig. 12.1 which is characterised by frequency and wavelength. This ranges from light, through radiowaves, X-rays and high-energy gamma radiation which is released in large quantities from a nuclear detonation. It should be noted that exposure to gamma radiation does not make something radioactive. Gamma radiation can travel many kilometres in air at the speed of light. It causes damage to tissues both internally and externally with both acute and delayed effects.

12.4.3   Particle Radiation

As the name suggested this type of radiation consists of subatomic or groups of subatomic particles. Three sorts are recognised: alpha, beta and neutrons. These and gamma radiation are termed ionising radiation.

12.4.3.1   Alpha Particles

Alpha particles are heavy and positively charged and contain two protons and two neutrons. They have a very short range in air but deposit large amounts of energy. They are blocked by intact skin and paper. If an alpha source (e.g. ^{210} Polonium) is ingested, it causes severe damage to the intestine and bone marrow.

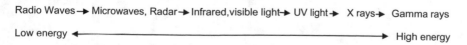

Radio Waves ➔ Microwaves, Radar ➔ Infrared,visible light ➔ UV light ➔ X rays ➔ Gamma rays

Low energy ◄――――――――――――――――――――――――――――――► High energy

Fig. 12.1 Spectrum of electromagnetic radiation

12.4.3.2   Beta Particles

Beta particles are small, negatively charged particles (electrons) which are released from decaying nuclei of a radioactive material. Beta particles can travel only a few metres in air. Irradiation of the skin by beta particles causes burns. The eye is also very vulnerable, leading to cataract formation.

12.4.3.3   Neutrons

These are uncharged particles which can travel many metres in air and pass through body tissues depositing large amounts of energy. They cause damage by the formation of ions which then react with molecules in the tissue. Neutrons are produced as a result of nuclear fission as in the detonation of a nuclear device.

12.4.4   The Measurement of Radiation

The German physician Roentgen originally studied the deposition of energy from X-rays in air and gave his name to the first unit used to measure radiation. Nowadays radiation is described in terms of the energy it releases when in contact with tissues. The original term used for this was the rad, but this has more recently been replaced by the Gray.

$$100\,\text{rads} = I\,\text{Joule}/\text{Kg of absorbed energy}$$

$$1\,\text{Gray}\,(\text{Gy}) = 100\,\text{rads}$$

Most exposures to radiation are small and thus the Centigray is often used to describe these (I Centigray = 1 rad).

12.4.4.1   Biological Equivalence

Because absorbed radiation creates different degrees of damage in different tissues absorbed doses of radiation are often expressed in rem (rads equivalent man) to allow for such differences. The rem has now been replaced officially by the Sievert (100 rem = I Sievert).

12.4.5   Radioactivity

Radioactivity is a property of a substance which releases radiation, both electro-magnetic and particulate. Such substances are usually termed radioisotopes. They are designated by their atomic weight e.g. Cobalt 60, used in radiotherapy which is known as ^{60}Co. The difference between radioactive isotopes and stable elements is that the former are releasing energy to achieve stability. Radioactivity is therefore a progressive process where one isotope is transformed into another and finally into a stable element that is no longer radioactive. An example already quoted is Polonium 210 which gradually changes into lead over a period of time determined by its half-life. Radioactivity is exponential and not linear and the reduction of radioactivity with time is described by the half-life. This is the time taken for the radioactivity of a specific quantity of radioisotope to reduce by half (see Box 12.5).

Box 12.5 Measurement of radioactivity
Radioactivity is measured by the number of disintegrations of the atoms within a radioisotope producing its characteristic radiation signature
  Key terms:
  Radioactive decay: the process by which radioactive isotopes emit radi-ation. Each isotope has a characteristic decay pattern in terms of the type of radiation emitted and its half-life
  Half-life: defined as the time required for half the atoms in a radioisotope to decay. Half-lives range from tiny fractions of a second to tens of thousands of years. The release of radioisotopes with long half-lives is associated with significant environmental contamination and risk to health.
  Radioactivity is measured in terms of the number of disintegrations per second. The first unit used was the Curie, which described 3.7×10^7 disin-tegrations per second. This proved to be too large for practical use and radioactivity was therefore usually expressed as milliCuries (mC) (10^6 mC = 1 Curie)
  More recently, the Curie has been replaced by the Bequerel (Bq) which is equivalent to one disintegration per second. This is however too small for practical use and kilo or mega Bq are usually used.

It is important to understand the difference between radiation (as defined above) and radioactivity. A radioisotope is characterised by its atomic weight and by the type and energy of the radiation it emits. Each radioisotope has a characteristic signature that helps detection and identification.

It is the radiation emitted from radioisotopes that causes trauma to the body. This can be prevented (1) by increasing the distance from the radioactive source and (2) by shielding the source with a heavy metal such as lead which absorbs radiation; shielding a source does not change its characteristic radioactivity but prevents it from escaping. The containment of a toxic chemical agent is a good analogy. Radioactivity from an isotope that is contaminating the surface of the body can also be reduced by decontamination (removal of the isotope) which also parallels contamination by a toxic chemical.

12.4.6   Key Points to Remember About Radiation and Radioactivity

- Radioactive contamination can only be produced by contact with a radioisotope in a form (e.g. a powder) that sticks to the body or is inhaled or ingested.
- Persons cannot be 'contaminated' by radiation (for example patients are not radioactive after having an X-ray)
- A person who is contaminated externally by a radioisotope can contaminate another person by contact (cf transmission of a persistent chemical hazard such as sulphur mustard). Radioactive contamination is therefore transmissible either from person to person or from a contaminated surface to a person. This poses a hazard to emergency responders
- Radioactive substances can enter the body also by inhalation or ingestion. This gives rise to internal radioactive contamination.

12.4.7   Exposure to Radiation and Radioactive Contamination: Prevention and Management

We have already noted that persons can be exposed to electromagnetic radiation without being radioactively contaminated. Contamination by a radioisotope can cause both external and internal radiation depending on whether or not the isotope has been ingested or inhaled. Internal contamination by an alpha emitting isotope is potentially very serious. Although these substances cannot penetrate skin they can penetrate the intestinal wall and the lung tissue. In doing so they deposit high levels of energy and cause serious damage to vulnerable body systems particularly the intestine and bone marrow.

12.4.7.1   Irradiation and Radioactive Contamination

Key points:
External irradiation
External irradiation occurs when the whole or part of the body is exposed from an external source (either from a nuclear explosion, with the release of gamma radiation, a reactor meltdown or exposure to a radioactive isotope).

The degree of injury caused depends on the dose of radiation received (measured in rads, rem or Sieverts). The dose of radiation received is defined as exposure time x exposure rate.

During exposure, radiation may pass completely through the body or be partially absorbed by the tissues.

Accidental exposure to a highly radioactive source such as ^{60}Co can affect the whole body but the greatest risk is to limited areas such as the hands from handling unprotected sources.

External radioactive contamination

External radioactive contamination occurs when a radioactive isotope (e.g. debris from a nuclear explosion) is deposited on the skin and clothing. Such debris is usually in the form of a dust. This contamination can be removed by surface cleaning with soap and water (as for chemical contamination). Care must be taken during external decontamination to avoid accidental ingestion and subsequent internal contamination.

Internal radioactive contamination

Internal radioactive contamination occurs when radioactive materials are inhaled, ingested or absorbed through open wounds. Internal contamination is more dangerous that external since particles such as alpha and low energy beta particles which do not penetrate the skin can easily penetrate the gut wall causing local damage and radiation injury to the bone marrow. The isotope ^{137}I which is a major product of nuclear explosions is concentrated after internal contamination in the thyroid thus exposing the gland to radiation injury. Giving iodine in such cases dilutes the accumulating radioactive iodine and reduces the local radioactivity in the gland.

12.4.7.2 Prevention of Exposure to Radiation

The penetration of radiation into the body depends on the type of radiation present. Charged particles (alpha and beta) are easily stopped (alpha particles cannot penetrate the skin). However, neutrons and gamma radiation can easily penetrate the body tissues as well as glass and plastic.

There are three key factors which provide protection against radiation injury

(1) Time of exposure.
The shorter the period spent near the radiation source the less will be the radiation dose received

(2) Distance from the source
The further away from the source of radiation, the less will be the dose received (the effects of radiation diminish with the square of the distance from the source)

(3) Shielding
Neutrons and gamma radiation have much diminished penetration of high-density materials such as lead and concrete. Providing shielding with

these materials greatly reduces the dose of radiation received. Thus radioisotopes used in everyday medical and industrial practice (e.g. ^{60}Co) are transported in lead containers. As with chemical hazards, if the hazard is contained the risk of danger from exposure is minimalised.

12.4.8   Injury from Radiological and Nuclear Agents

Injury from R and N agents can broadly be classified according to likelihood and severity as follows:

Least likely-most harmful: most likely-least harmful

12.4.8.1   Causes of Radiation Injury

(1) Detonation of a nuclear weapon
(2) Meltdown of a nuclear reactor. This involves overheating and melting of the nuclear fuel rods with the subsequent, possible explosive release of radioactive material. It should be noted that the explosion in this case is not nuclear but related to the reactor cooling system. The reactor failures in Chernobyl in the Ukraine and at Fukushima in Japan are examples. Both produced the release of high concentrations of radioactive isotopes.
(3) The deliberate explosive dispersal of a radioactive isotope This is termed a radioactive dispersal device and consists of a conventional explosive device surrounded by a radioactive material. The device is a potential terrorist threat and is popularly known as a 'dirty bomb'.
(4) Accidental release or inappropriate disposal of radioactive substances

Accidental exposures to radioactivity have occurred when radioisotopes used in hospital radiotherapy or for industrial purposes have been disposed with general waste without suitable protection. In addition to accidental exposure, radioactivity has also been used in homicidal attacks as demonstrated by the poisoning of Alexander Litvinenko in London in 2006 by the radioisotope Polonium 210.

12.4.9   The Trauma of Ionising Radiation

Radiation causes injury to the body in three ways:

(1) Focal tissue damage and necrosis. This occurs when a radioactive source is in close contact with the skin.
(2) Acute radiation sickness. This occurs after exposure to high levels of radiation. The clinical presentation depends on the radiation dose absorbed. There are

Table 12.1 The Nature and timing of signs and symptoms of the acute radiation syndrome

Early symptoms	Time of onset after exposure	Radiation dose	Final radiation trauma effects
Nausea, vomiting	Within 48 h	100 rad (1 Gy)	Decrease in white cells and platelets
Nausea, vomiting	Within 24 h	200 rad (2 Gy)	Marked decrease in white cells and platelets (haemopoietic syndrome
Nausea, vomiting and diarrhoea	Within 8 h	400 rad (4 Gy)	Damage to the small intestine (50 % mortality in the absence of treatment
Nausea, vomiting and diarrhoea	Within 5 min	1000–3000 rad (10–30 Gy)	Severe gastrointestinal damage. Very poor prognosis
Change in mental status, fitting	Within a few minutes	>3000 rad (>30 Gy)	Severe CNS damage with cardiovascular collapse. Lethal

three essential phases of acute radiation syndrome: (1) prodromal, (2) latent period and (3) manifest illness

(3) Long-term effects. Radiation affects the DNA of the cells and can cause mutations in the structure. This can lead to the production of cancerous neoplasms e.g. leukaemia

The effects of whole body irradiation cause a group of syndromes which are known collectively as acute radiation syndrome (ARS). It should be noted that ARS only occurs after whole body and not localised irradiation. The nature and the timing of signs and symptoms of ARS are dependent on the dose received. In general, the higher the dose received and the earlier the signs and symptoms occur the worse the prognosis. Table 12.1 lists the signs and symptoms of ARS as a function of dose.

12.5 Comparison of the Trauma Produced by Chemical, Biological, Radiological and Nuclear Agents

Chemical, biological, radiological and nuclear agents, despite being classed together produce very different types of trauma. This is related to the key properties of each agent which may be related to those discussed in Chap. 3 for chemical hazards.

These are as follows:

(1) Physical form and properties of the agent
(2) Persistency—how long the agent will remain in the environment
(3) Toxicity—how the agent causes trauma to the body
(4) Latency—the time taken for physical signs and symptoms to appear

12.5.1 Physical Form

(1) Chemical agents. The physical form of chemical hazards was discussed in Sect. 3.6.1.
(2) Biological agents. Bacteria may survive in or out of the body depending on whether they can form spores (e.g. anthrax). Viruses are dependent on invading the cell and using the intracellular apparatus for their survival. Both bacteria and viruses are very susceptible to physical factors when outside the body host (e.g. heat and light)
(3) Radiological agents. Radioisotopes may exist in solid, dust or liquid forms. They are resistant to the normal environmental factors.
(4) Nuclear agents consist of solid highly radioactive materials which are found in nuclear weapons or in nuclear reactors in the form of metallic fuel rods (e.g. ^{235}U).

12.5.2 Persistency

Chemical
The persistency of chemical agents was discussed in Sect. 3.6.2. The concept provides a model for both biological and radiological hazards

Biological
The ability of pathogenic organisms to live outside a human or animal host is very variable. The normal method of transmission is by insect, animal and human vectors. Bacteria and viruses can be kept alive under laboratory conditions but in the open air they are very vulnerable to weather and other environmental conditions. Sunlight for example rapidly degrades bacteria in an aerosol as a biological weapon. The AIDS virus is very susceptible outside the human host and does not survive for more than a few minutes. However some bacteria (e.g. anthrax) can form spores which can remain in the environment for many years. When in contact with a normal host they rapidly change from spores to their normal infectious form. During the second world war British scientists deliberately distributed anthrax spores in the small uninhabited island of Gruinard in Scotland. The spores remained in the ground for more than forty years and the island finally had to be decontaminated by removing all the top soil and destroying the spores by heating.

Radiological
As noted above, the radioactivity produced by a radioisotope is described in terms of its half-life. The persistency of a radiation hazard therefore is a function of this and also the physical form in which the isotope is distributed. Radioisotopes can exist in gas, liquid or sold form. The radioactive gas Radon is naturally released at low levels into the atmosphere from granitic rocks. Radioactive isotopes dispersed as a dust can create a highly persistent contamination whose hazard then depends

on the half-life. Radioactive fallout from a nuclear detonation contains isotopes with very long half-lives (e.g. strontium 90). A radiation dispersal device which might be used by terrorists can leave similar radioactive contamination with a long duration (e.g. Cobalt 60). Note that the explosion which causes this dispersal is from a conventional high explosive and not from nuclear fission.

Nuclear

The explosion of a nuclear weapon causes both physical and radiation injury. There is immediate release of non-persistent high-energy gamma radiation and neutrons. If the bomb is detonated at ground level a radioactive dust cloud forms which can produce highly persistent radioactive contamination determined by the half-lives of the products involved. These are often very long, lasting up to thousands of years.

12.5.3 Toxicity

We have seen earlier in the book that toxicity is what an agent does to the body to cause harm. Section 3.6.3 noted that this is a function of dose for chemical agents and this maxim can be extended to biological, radiological and nuclear agents.

(1) Chemical

The concept of toxicity of chemical substances was discussed in Chap. 3 and can be expressed as LD_{50} or LCt_{50} if the toxic chemical is inhaled

(2) Biological

Bacteria cause damage to the body cells and organs by producing toxins which are essentially chemical in nature (Chap. 11). Thus toxic trauma is the final pathway of bacterial infection. For biological agents the effectiveness of an agent in causing an infection is described in terms of the number of bacteria required to establish infection. Unlike bacteria, viruses cause damage to the body by taking over the cellular apparatus and using it for their self-replication. This disrupts cellular metabolism and genetic control.

(3) Radiological

Radioisotopes cause damage to the body cells from both local and whole body exposure. Toxicity to the body cells is caused by ionising radiation which has chemical final pathways disrupting cellular metabolism and also genetic control. The latter can produce mutations of cells that can lead to neoplasms, for example leukaeumia. This genetic damage can be compared with the chemical agent sulphur mustard which is also known to be carcinogenic.

(4) Nuclear

The detonation of a nuclear weapons produces severe physical and thermal injury. In addition, there is also radiation trauma from the radiation of the detonation and also from the released radioactive isotopes.

12.5.4   Latency

(1) Chemical
   The wide range of time intervals for the appearance of toxic trauma, known as latency was discussed for chemical agents in Sect. 3.6.4. The same dose of a toxic agent will produce effects at different times in a human or animal population which is described by a normal distribution.

(2) Biological
   For bacteria and viruses, the concept of latency in normal infection is familiar as the incubation period. This is usually days to weeks. Importantly, the latent period for biological agents is considerably longer overall than for chemical agents. This is important if BW agents are used in a civil setting where detection capabilities are limited and confirmation of an attack comes from clusters of presenting signs and symptoms. Latency is therefore a major consideration in deciding whether a possible terrorist attack has been chemical or biological.

(3) Radiological
   As mentioned previously, radiation injury is dose dependent. Following a prodromal phase in acute radiation sickness, there is a latent period of several days before the development of radiation syndromes.

(4) Nuclear
   The physical trauma following a nuclear blast is ultra short and the injury pattern immediately recognisable. Immediate radiation effects following exposure to high dose radiation are visible within minutes to hours as described in Sect. 12.4.9.

12.5.5   Protection and Decontamination

The correct level of protection against C, B, R and N agents is an important consideration. Each class of agent requires very different levels of protection. Not all agents require the high level of personal protection afforded by level A self-contained protective suits. A good example of appropriate protection levels was illustrated by the large number of 'white powder' incidents following the deliberate release of anthrax spores in the USA in 2001. Many of these incidents were hoaxes but in most countries the emergency responders chose to wear the highest level of CBRN protection (level A) which is not appropriate for a biological agent attack. Putting on this level of protection takes considerable time and exposes the wearer to a number of risks which are not appropriate for the level of danger posed by the hazard.

Similarly, there are considerable differences in decontamination requirements for individual C, B, R and N agents.

(1) Chemical

Chapter 4 presented the graded levels of personal protection appropriate for the different classes of chemical released. It also discussed the decontamination of persistent agents. It is important to realise that not all chemical agents are persistent as is the case with many biological agents.

(2) Biological

Overall, for biological agents the level of protection required, both for the skin and the respiratory routes is less than that required for chemical agents. Following the release of a biological agent, or during management of a natural epidemic, protection is required (1) for direct inhalational exposure to an aerosol containing the agent and also direct inhalational contact with infected patients (2) against liquid contamination from body fluids. Such a level of protection is achieved using a light biological level C suit and HEPA filtration masks. The rules of operation in a biologically contaminated area are the same as those for hospital infection. The recent outbreak of Ebola in West Africa provides a good example of such procedures in dealing with a highly infectious and dangerous pathogen.

Personal protective ensembles for chemical agents are effective against biological agents also. Military filtration respirators are designed to cope with both classes of hazard. Level C protection is the most suitable or level D with light protective gloves.

Decontamination of biological agents follows the same principles as for chemical agents using standard disinfecting agents (e.g. bleach).

(3) Radiation and radioactivity protection.

Radiation does not contaminate a person whereas a radioactive isotope can. Personal protection is therefore not required in managing a patient who has been irradiated. However protection is required when there is obvious or suspected contamination by a radioisotope. Protection against a radiation source is provided by physical protection as in concrete shelters or by increasing the distance from the source and decreasing the time spent in a radioactive area. The degree of personal protection required against a contaminated patient is therefore appropriate to protect against physical contamination by radioactive dust. PPE will not provide protection against gamma radiation and neutrons but it does provide protection against alpha and beta particle radiation.

Decontamination of radioactive substances is achieved by physical removal and also washing with soap and water. The effluent produced is of course radioactive and must be contained and removed rather than allowed to run into drainage systems.

12.6   Conclusions

Chemical, biological, radiological and nuclear agents are classed together as CBRN agents and are often termed 'weapons of mass destruction.' This term is misleading and is not accurate in the medical sense, where appropriate and early treatment of mass casualties can prevent mass fatalities. CBRN agents have certain characteristics in common, such as toxicity, latency and persistency but cause harm to the body in different ways. An understanding of the properties of chemical, biological, and radiation-producing substances is essential to the prevention of trauma and the correct management of casualties.

Suggestions for Further Reading

Alibek A (2000) Biohazard. Arrow books. Random House Group, London
Briggs SM (2014) (ed) Advanced disaster medical response manual for providers. Cine-Med Publishing Ltd, Woodbury
Centers for Disease Control and Prevention (2016) Bioterrorism Agents. Available at http://emergency.cdc.gov/agent/agentlist.asp. Accessed 15 March 2016
Cocciardi JA (2004) Weapons of mass destruction and terrorism response—a field guide. Jones and Bartlett, Sudbury
Paxman J, Harris R (2002) A higher form of killing. Arrow books. Random House Group, London
UK Department of Health CBRN Handbook (2008) Available at https://www.gov.uk/.../chemical-biological-radiological-and-nuclear-incidents-recognise-and-respond. Accessed 05 March 2016

Appendices

Appendix A: Physical Characteristics of Common Toxic Industrial Chemicals

Chemical	UN HAZMAT ID number	Latency	Persistency	Toxicity threshold (ppm/h) impairment/fatality	Odour
Allyl alcohol	1098	S	L	7.7/22	Mustard-like
Acrolein	1092	S	I	0.1/1.4	1 ppm acrid and sweet
Acrylonitrile	1093	S	I	35/75	17 ppm unpleasant peach-like
Ammonia	1005	S	S	110/1100	17 ppm sharp suffocating
Arsine	2188	S–L	I	0.2/0.5	0.5 ppm garlic
Chlorine	1017	S I	S–I	3/22	Pungent (bleach)
Diborane	1911	S	I	1/15	2.5 ppm sweet
Ethylene oxide	2983	S	I	45/200	425 ppm ether-like
Formaldehyde	1078	S	L	10/25	1 ppm characteristic pungent
Hydrogen bromide	1048	S	I	3/30	2 ppm pungent, stinging
Hydrogen chloride	2186	S	I	22/104	0.77 ppm pungent, irritating
Hydrogen cyanide	1051/1641	S	S	7/15–50	1–5 ppm characteristic bitter almond
Hydrogen fluoride	1790	S–L	I	22/44	0.4 ppm sharp, irritating
Hydrogen selenide	2202	S	S–I	0.2/1.5	0.3 ppm horseradish
Hydrogen sulphide	1053	S–L	S–I	30/100	0.1 ppm characteristic rotten eggs
Methyl hydrazine	1244	S–L	L	1/3	1 ppm ammonia-like

(continued)

© Springer International Publishing Switzerland 2016
D.J. Baker, *Toxic Trauma*, DOI 10.1007/978-3-319-40916-0

231

(continued)

Chemical	UN HAZMAT ID number	Latency	Persistency	Toxicity threshold (ppm/h) impairment/fatality	Odour
Hydrazine	2030	S–L	L	13/35	3 ppm ammonia-like
Methyl isocyanate	2480	S	I	0.5/5	2 ppm pungent
Methyl mercaptan	1064	S	I	5/23	0.002 ppm rotten cabbage (at 1 ppm odour fatigue begins)
Nitrogen dioxide	1067	L	I	12/20	?1 ppm pungent
Nitric acid	1760	S	L	4/22	1 ppm characteristic choking, acrid
Parathion	1967	S–L	S–I	0.2/0.8	0.4 ppm
Phosgene	1076	S–L	S–I	0.3/5	0.5 ppm characteristic new mown hay
Phosphine	2199	S–L	I	0.3/1.1–30	0.9 ppm characteristic rotten fish
Sulphuric acid	1830	S	L	2.5/7.5	Odourless (sulphur dioxide smell when heated)
Sulphur dioxide	1079	S–L	I	3/15–100	1 ppm characteristic coke fumes
Toluene di-isocyanate	2078	S	L	0.08/0.51	0.4–2 ppm pungent

Key Latency: Short = minutes to hours, Long = hours to days. Persistency: Short = minutes to hours, Intermediate = hours to days, Long = days to weeks
Information source US Army Center for Health Promotion and Preventative Medicine. *Industrial Chemical Prioritization and Determination of Critical Hazards of Concern*. Aberdeen Proving Ground, Md: USACHPPM; 2003: Appendix B. USACHPPM Report 47–EM–6154–03 *S* short, *L* long, *I* intermediate

Appendix B: Physical Characteristics of the Major Chemical Warfare and Riot Control Agents

Agent class	Agent	Freezing point (°C)	Boiling point	Physical state at 20 °C	Vapour density	Odour
Lung-damaging agents	Chlorine	−101	−34	Gas	2.45	Pungent
	Phosgene	−118	+8.2	Gas	3.4	New mown hay
	Diphosgene	−57	+127	Liquid and vapour	6.9	Green apples
	Methyl isocyanate[a]		+39.1	Gas	0.96	

(continued)

(continued)

Agent class	Agent	Freezing point (°C)	Boiling point	Physical state at 20 °C	Vapour density	Odour
Nerve agents	Tabun (GA)	−49	+240	Liquid	5.63	Fruity
	Sarin (GB)	−56	+147	Liquid	4.86	Fruity
	Soman (GD)	−70	+167	Liquid	6.33	Fruity
	VX	−30	+300	Liquid	9.2	
Chemical asphyxiants	Hydrogen cyanide	−13.9	+26.5	Liquid and vapour	0.93	Almonds
	Cyanogen chloride	−6	+12.5	Liquid	2.1	Almonds
Vesicants	Sulphur mustard gas	+14.5	+227.8	Liquid and vapour	5.4	Garlic or mustard
	Lewisite	−13	+190	Liquid and vapour	7.2	Geraniums
Incapacitating agents	BZ	+165		White powder		
Respiratory irritant (riot control agents)	CS	+95	+310	White powder		Pungent
	CR	+72		Pale yellow powder		

Nerve agents all have a freezing point below zero and are in the liquid state at an ambient temperature of 20 °C. Although they all boil above 100 °C, all except VX exhibit a significant vapour pressure. VX therefore poses less of an inhalational risk than the others but is more persistent. Agents that are gases at ambient temperature are very volatile and therefore non-persistent. Incapacitating and irritant agents all have a very high-freezing point and are solids at ambient temperature. They are dispersed in a pulverized form in aerosols. With the exception of hydrogen cyanide, the agents listed above have a vapour density greater than air. They therefore tend to concentrate immediately above the ground. Odour is not a physical property but is included here since it has provided an important early warning of chemical agent release since the First World War. Only impure nerve agents have a characteristic fruity odour noted above

[a]Methyl isocyanate is not a CW agent but has caused mass inhalational injury and is included in comparison with the CW lung-damaging agents

Index

© Springer International Publishing Switzerland 2016
D.J. Baker, *Toxic Trauma*, DOI 10.1007/978-3-319-40916-0

Printed in the United States
By Bookmasters